# Quantified

# Quantified

## Biosensing Technologies in Everyday Life

edited by Dawn Nafus

The MIT Press
Cambridge, Massachusetts
London, England

This book was set in Sabon by the MIT Press. Printed and bound in the United States of America.

Library of Congress Cataloging-in-Publication Data

Names: Nafus, Dawn, editor.
Title: Quantified : biosensing technologies in everyday life / Nafus, Dawn, ed.
Other titles: Biosensing technologies in everyday life
Description: Cambridge, MA : The MIT Press, [2016] | Includes bibliographical references and index.
Identifiers: LCCN 2015038388| ISBN 9780262034173 (hardcover : alk. paper) | ISBN 9780262528757 (pbk. : alk. paper)
Subjects: | MESH: Biosensing Techniques. | Confidentiality. | Monitoring, Physiologic--trends.
Classification: LCC R857.B54 | NLM QT 36.4 | DDC 610.28/4--dc23 LC record available at http://lccn.loc.gov/2015038388

10 9 8 7 6 5 4 3 2 1

# Contents

# Acknowledgments

First I would like to thank the contributors to this book, whose collaborative spirit ensured this work came to light. In particular, the participants in the Biosensors in Everyday Life program have been excellent partners to think with. Nina Wakeford and Joanna Wilkinson made invaluable contributions to that program, and their presence is visible, to me at least, in these pages. At Intel, Suzanne Thomas, David Gordon, Margie Morris, Mic McGrath, Mic Bowman, Henry Gabb, Mike Wrinn, Richard Beckwith, ken anderson, and John Sherry have all provided valuable support, advice, and debate throughout the stages of this project. Intel's University Research Office provided the financial support necessary to accomplish much of the research in these pages. The Data Sense team—Lama Nachman, Pete Denman, Sangita Sharma, Evan Savage, Rita Wouhaybi, Lenitra Durham, Devon Strawn, and Tim Coppernoll—taught me more about data and design than I ever thought possible and gave me a new perspective on what a contribution from the social sciences could be. Who knew filing bug reports could be so rewarding? Collaborative Design MFA students at Pacific Northwest College of Art clarified the concept of this book with their sharp questions, and Bryce Peake took the idea of anthropological research through building to a whole new level. Melissa Cefkin demonstrated by example the kinds of intellectual contributions that can be made from an industrial setting, and James Leach, Bill Graves, Carrie Humphrey, and Lisa Nakamura provided mentorship early in my career that made this work possible. Within the Quantified Self community, Anne Wright, Steven Jonas, and Robin Barooah were amazing guides and educators. Gary Wolf and Ernesto Ramirez deserve special thanks for giving us anthropologists so much to talk about.

Finally, I'd especially like to thank Gina Neff for giving me the kick in the pants I needed to start on this work, Margy Avery for shepherding its early phases, and Gita Manaktala for seeing it through. I owe much more than can be expressed here to my parents, Penni and Jim Nafus, who deserve tremendous credit for their patient support. Last, but certainly not least, my dear partner Dan Jaffee provided incredibly generous feedback and eagle-eyed suggestions, amongst things.

# Introduction

Dawn Nafus

## A Critical Encounter

My first encounter with biosensing was in 2009, when a colleague ran some ideas past me for research projects he thought promising. While I maintain my own scholarly commitments as an anthropologist, and publish in the normal academic way, I do not work at a university but inside the research and development labs of Intel, a large computer hardware company.[1] Most of these ideas were technical research topics worthy of computer science dissertations, such as how indoor location sensing could be made more precise. Another one of the proposed projects involved something my colleague called "biosensors," which he explained are a special class of computer components called "sensors" designed to detect various bodily phenomena, such as perspiration rates, or the levels of glucose or oxygen in blood. Biosensors take signals from these things and turn them into electronic data. He had seen the technical trajectory for biosensors—they were getting smaller and cheaper, just as computers had gone from mainframes to PCs. Because miniaturization had enabled computing to go from an expert-only affair to everyday use by nonengineers, he projected that biosensors would similarly no longer be limited to large medical labs with large budgets. An ordinary person could buy one. Would they want to, though, or was this a mere flight of industry fancy? If mass adoption of personal biosensors were to happen, the commercial implications could be enormous—not just for Intel, but also for many firms across a variety of industries.

I thought about it. The implications sent shivers down my spine. Being somewhat familiar with the basic lessons of medical anthropology, and even more familiar with the ways that expert forms of knowledge have become tools of social control by subjecting anything and everything to quantification, whether appropriate or not, this seemed like a spectacularly bad idea. To my mind the implication was a clear probability that these technologies would exacerbate this deeply problematic form of social control. It is a job requirement to speak up when I have reason to believe either that there is no market for the technologies under consideration, or that the social risks and institutional costs of entering that market make it a poor idea. This seemed to clearly fall into the latter category, and I was prepared to tell him so.

I remember that a now-embarrassing smugness came over me in this moment. I resembled the breed of critic Latour (2004) so roundly lampoons, who revels in showing the naïve believers in a technology that "whatever [the believers] think, their behavior is entirely determined by the action of powerful causalities coming from objective reality they don't see [social structure, power, etc.], but that you, yes you, the never sleeping critic, alone can see" (239). In truth, I wanted nothing more than to give my colleague an earful about panopticality and Foucault, but my experience had been that delivering earfuls rarely ends well. Instead I appealed to empiricism. I explained how the predecessors to these technologies—bathroom scales—in fact have not succeeded in "encouraging" people to lose weight, but more often simply add to the intense guilt, shame, and anxiety people already have about their bodies. The Foucauldians would note that that is the point to such things—that social control happens not just by legal fiat or physical violence, but also by the capacity to convince people to see themselves only through the lens of what the more powerful would see (here, the narrow band of "normal" weight, now statistically abnormal in the United States but defined as "normal" by the medical profession). This well-established technique of social control works by compelling people to take on the task of controlling their bodies according to the categories that others produce, as if it were one's own idea all along.

It would be fair to say that the issue was not merely an intellectual one. The very question of whether there was social or market value in biosensing technologies summoned in me the toxic combination of shame and anger I too feel when I am subjected to such "encouragements" about my body. I recalled the patronizing tone a nurse once took with me about how a "woman of your age should really be taking folic acid," without the faintest knowledge of the contents of my uterus or the painful social costs I pay for my reproductive choices. I began to imagine the horror of being sent a text message about how fat I would no doubt get if my various biosensor readings didn't change, all because a thinnish white man in Silicon Valley took it upon himself to solve the obesity crisis,[2] and offered a mobile phone-based solution that effectively turned a complex social phenomenon with deep-rooted structural causes into my personal responsibility to solve. I might live with such a technology for a few days, at which point I would enthusiastically throw it out the window, most likely straight after a proper dessert. With port.

Having mulled over these things, I told my colleague that these new biosensors are much more likely to do harm than good. I asked whether he really wanted to go into a market where actual utility is likely to be so low, and risks so high. Frankly, I didn't see reason to sponsor university research on the topic, if the answer was so obvious and clear.

"Okay, I see your point about the guilt and anxiety," he responded. "But I am a diabetic. If I don't know my glucose level, I could die. How is that not useful?"

I had to concede the point.

What we ultimately agreed was that there was a set of empirical and theoretical questions here that required closer examination. Our answer was going to be found in the complexities and contingencies of social life, not in any claims about the utility (or lack thereof) of a particular product to a particular individual, which is what market research traffics in. It was not a problem that market research could handle, but one that raised intensely challenging social questions that only scholarship could meaningfully pursue. Figuring out whether a consumer market for biosensors was even thinkable had everything to do with whether the data they produced cohered with a cultural and social imaginary, such that users stood a chance of making sense of them. It had to do with whether socially productive design strategies were conceivable, or whether the social systems made the conditions of possibility for these technologies a dead end.

This book, then, has its origins in a controversy that shows no sign of abating. The temporary agreement with my colleague eventually became the Biosensors in Everyday Life program, a three-year program involving four universities, which provided space for us to continue our discussion with more evidence. All of the projects from that program are represented in this volume, alongside others.[3] Time has answered my colleague's question about whether a consumer market is feasible—ninety million wearable sensors were shipped globally in 2014 (ABI 2014), most of which are designed to sense the body. The underlying reason for the debate between us has not simply resolved itself. Nor will it. Biosensors mediate uncertain, sometimes fraught relations between medical practice and self-care, between scientific knowledge and lay knowledge, between community and commercial impulses, and between aesthetic production and instrumentality. They represent a significant new chapter in the ongoing story of what it is that numbers do for us, and do to us. Who gets to enumerate their bodily experiences—and who is begrudgingly made to do so? Enumeration can mobilize the cultural logic of numbers as abstractions, as claims to superior truth, but it also can mobilize the equally long history of enumeration as an embodied, situated practice. Are these numbers a mere tool of capitalist accumulation, or participatory knowledge making that cannot be understood in those terms? Is privacy truly dead, a fantasy that never was, or a right that must be asserted anew?

These are all high-stakes questions. As these devices continue to proliferate, they could yet become the very worst modernity has to offer—social control masquerading as science, and the soulless abstraction of bodies into bits, to name two ugly prospects—or they could participate in a flourishing of alternatives. There are still collective choices to make about what social logics will be mobilized, and we cannot afford to think about these technologies as finished products awaiting after-the-fact comment. Technologies are never a done deal, and this book aims to reopen the negotiations, so to speak. With less desirable paradigms in such strong positions of power, shaping these technologies into something better than the current offerings requires a tremendous amount of work, however necessary.

This is also work that requires a more expansive notion of critique. The ability to see outside of one's current position is perhaps the only way to imagine how things might be otherwise, yet the cartoonish critic-denouncer role I initially played has little to offer those who would begin crafting, imagining, and, yes, physically building alternatives. Here I draw inspiration from Latour's version of the critic, who "is not the one who lifts the rug from under the feet of the naïve believers, but the one who offers the participants arenas in which to gather" (2004, 246). This book is designed to be that sort of arena, socially situated in its own way but committed to enabling the broadest possible participation in the discussion of what biosensing could come to mean. It includes views from the social sciences and cultural studies, and from those who are primarily concerned with "convening" materials together into physical or digital objects.

This volume is intended to serve as a resource to inform conversations like the one I found myself in, wherever social choices about biosensors are being made. I say "choice" as a way to acknowledge the very real power many of us have to reshape our material world, including those of us without formal positions or large budgets. "Choice" is a term that has its problems, but it reminds us that the direction of our material world is not inevitable, and that readers of this book are part of its shaping. I do not say "choice" to elide the important experiences of those who have no meaningful choice when biosensing is foisted upon them, such as when an employer requires its employees to wear physical activity monitors. As chapter 5 points out, it is important that we always acknowledge when there is no neoliberal "choosing" one's way out of such a situation. Choices are also not limited to deliberative democratic processes, or the kinds of societies that choose policies through participatory discussion and debate. The choices I have in mind involve difficult struggles and frequent failures where social realities fall far short of open deliberation. The social and technical arrangements we live with will be decided in public outcries, in legislative changes, and in the hands-on, painstaking work of building hardware and calculating data. They will be decided through changes in policies by companies, governments, and research institutions, and in the ad-hoc practices of those who work for them. And, of course, they will emerge through the quotidian exchange between technology user and technology developer, and the cascade of adjustments to material infrastructures necessary to support the continued use of these technologies. Each is an important moment in the unfolding of this new technology, and in each, choices will be made, deliberatively or not, based on beliefs about what is within the sphere of conceivability.

A social scientific understanding of the kinds of social relations that are conceivable can, I believe, make a positive contribution to the public discussion by making more choices available. So can perspectives from people who build things, who can articulate, and expand, the material realities of what biosensors can and cannot do. This volume contains both perspectives. It unpacks what is at stake socially, culturally, politically, and economically when biosensors become a matter of lived everyday practice. It critically examines biosensing practices both as a new extension of social control, and as a site where alternative modalities of power are being forged. It exposes the intertwining of materiality, everyday practices, economic relations, communities, and new medical and legal formations that shape these new socio-technical practices.

## What Are These Things and Where Did They Come From?

For the purposes of this book, we focus on biosensing technologies, defined as technologies that indicate something about the body or the physical environment. If you ask an electrical engineer what a biosensor is, the definition she will give you will likely be more specific. A biosensor proper combines a biological element (like sweat, saliva, or CO2) with a physiochemical detector, often optical or electrochemical. The detector interacts with the substance being analyzed, and converts some aspect of it into an electrical signal. These sensors in turn form one part of much larger sensor systems, which include all the other components necessary to go from electrical signal to display on a screen or other type of communication. One reason biosensors are proliferating is that new techniques have been developed to use light for identifying ever more minute substances (see chapter 10 for an explanation of how these techniques work). If light can be used to detect the signatures of tiny substances, then the kinds of substances that can be discerned and turned into data grow exponentially. This expansion is what makes biosensors interesting from a social perspective.

From the perspective of an engineer, if you don't have liquid or gas touching a detector, you haven't got a biosensor. Sensors that detect movement do not count in this narrower definition. While this distinction matters deeply if you are trying to build a biosensor, it is not necessarily socially significant. A person using sensors to understand her patterns of stress may or may not care whether that stress is detected through cortisol levels in saliva using "wet" biosenors or the comparatively "dry" electroencephalogram (EEG). In this volume, we use the term "biosensing" to refer to any *practice* that uses information technology to understand something about bodies or the environments in which they live, whether the technology is at the cutting edge or not. This might involve a biosensor of the type already described. It might involve one of the many sensors currently ubiquitous in computers and mobile phones, used to indicate something about the body or the environment (e.g., accelerometers which detect movement in space, microphones and cameras, timers, GPS), but which are not, strictly speaking, biosensors. Finally, it might involve manually recording events (the foods one ate, the mood one was in, etc.) in a mobile phone application, in a spreadsheet, or on paper to varying levels of precision. Indeed, many biosensing services invite their users to manually record additional phenomena related to what the sensors sense. This perhaps says something interesting about the limitations of sensors. Sensors now capture more than ever, and more than their designers anticipated (often called "data exhaust"), but the human capacity to imagine what is meaningful to record necessarily exceeds sensors' capabilities.

This adaptation of an engineer's term has advantages. Focusing on biosensing foregrounds the sensors, and therefore the very physical link back to what is being sensed. This connection is important, and can easily be lost in a more data-centric view, especially one that focuses on the bigness of data accumulations. By examining biosensing practices, we can follow biosensors (proper) as a set of objects that change over time, yet have much in common with their predecessors, such as accelerometers. Wherever they might ultimately go, we can attend to the uncertainties they encounter in their travels.

There is a nascent but rapidly growing social scientific interest in the Quantified Self community,[4] in which biosensing enthusiasts meet in person to discuss what they have learned from their technologies. There is also growing social scientific interest in the "quantified self" phenomenon as constructed outside this community,[5] through idioms of datafication (van Dijck 2014), big data (Neff 2013), digital labor (Till 2014), self-surveillance (Lupton 2014a), and data doubles (Ruckenstein 2014). However, there is not yet social scientific work that focuses on biosensors as a class of technical objects; that is, other work largely prefigures which social phenomena the technologies engage with. Not all biosensing is about the quantified self, or about big data. As both Sherman and Taylor (chapters 2 and 9 in this volume) show, not all biosensor data are aggregated at great scale, nor does "bigness" capture everything that is, or could be, meaningful about this data. Nor is all biosensing about measuring selves. Indeed, in Böhlen's work on water-quality sensing in Indonesia (chapter 10), the self would be a wildly inappropriate starting point. Notions of the quantified self are hardly irrelevant to this volume; indeed, the person who coined the term, Gary Wolf, is the author of chapter 4. Although sensors always quantify, "the quantified self" is deliberately not the overall framing device of the book. The phrase is too apt; it taps too strongly into longstanding Western tropes of calculative rationality and preoccupations with the individual as the privileged locus of action. Instead, the focus on biosensing requires us to slow down our judgment about who is tracking what.[6] It opens up a view onto the diversity of practices possible by making it harder to pretend that we already know, by looking at the technology itself, what sort of phenomenon we are examining—a trap I clearly fell into in my first encounter with the topic.

The purposes to which these sensors are put are varied, and you will encounter many in the chapters to come. Devices designed for fitness monitoring (that count steps and measure distance run, heart rate, etc.) are easily seen on any street in North American or European cities. Medical and quasi-medical devices are less visible, but no less pervasive. Examples include glucose monitors, fertility monitors that track basal temperatures, implanted sensors to monitor the workings of the organs or contents of the blood, and devices that assess posture, or the sleeping position of an infant. There is an extensive literature on using sensors to remotely monitor the elderly (Mort et al. 2013; Mort, Roberts, and Callén 2013; Pols 2011). Because that literature is fairly well known, it has not been directly addressed in this volume, but it is notable that in many senses the predecessors to these technologies can be found in assisted living facilities. It is also notable that the elderly have proved as able to subvert the intentions of sensor system designers as their younger counterparts in the Quantified Self community who fancy themselves hackers and tinkers.

Finally, biosensors are being used to understand, and keep track of, the "-omes," not just genomes but also exposomes (the pollutants to which bodies are exposed) and microbiomes (the microbes in our bodies believed to affect physical and mental states). Consumer-grade environmental monitoring technologies are less robust and more expensive than those that grew out of medicine, but they too are getting smaller and cheaper. In genome and microbiome sensing, the sensing is conducted in a lab, and participants mail in samples. Accessing such data has become relatively simple, and thus these sensors raise the same social questions as a sensor worn on the wrist. In the "-omes," the sensing capabilities largely outpace the scientific understanding of the effects on the body of the substance being sensed. Indeed, in the case of the American Gut Project,[7] participants know that the data they receive back about their bodies in exchange for contributing to that research project may or may not be interpretable.

These sensors did not simply arrive on the market free of social entanglements. The fact that we often talk about technologies as asocial objects that need to be *set* in some context is itself evidence of the kind of context they are in (Strathern 2001)—one that considers them to be "free" of social origins. While a full genealogy of these technologies is impossible to trace here, I will pull on a few significant threads. Computation and medical knowledge have been intertwined since the 1960s (November 2012). The relation is most starkly visible in genomics research, where biologists use machine learning techniques to expand their statistical repertoire. However, it was the shift in computer science toward "ubiquitous computing" in the early 1990s (Weiser 1991) that set the stage for biomedicine's entry into popular use of computers. Ubiquitous computing is a vision in which the best computer is the one that becomes all but invisible to its user, moving off the desktop and into a computationally rich environment. While this vision cannot entirely be credited or blamed for all of what today's mobile phones, tablets, wearable computers, and smart buildings do, it has made the dispersion of computation beyond the PC conceivable. This dispersion created physical spaces on the body (pockets, wristbands) that were inhabitable by information technology, into which biosensors fit relatively easily.

Biosensors also cannot be understood outside the social history of biomedicalization, which Greenfield (chapter 7) and Kragh-Furbo et al. (chapter 1) address more deeply. I will only note here that biomedical ways of understanding the body have become inescapable in postindustrial societies. They have been inserted into ever more corners of social life. In that sense, it is thoroughly unsurprising that technologists have seen fit to turn their energies to building instruments of individual bodily control through the idiom of medical science. However, computer science and the information technology (IT) industry do not take all social changes surrounding them to be their cause (to wit: feminism), and so in that sense, the biomedicalization of information technologies was far from inevitable. One important mechanism by which biomedical frameworks became embedded in technical systems is through the subfield of "persuasive computing" (Fogg 2002). In this subfield, designers of technical systems abandoned a long-standing self-image of social neutrality, and set themselves the task of "nudging" their users toward the "right" behaviors, often by using the psychology of game design ("gamification," see Whitson 2013). While this acknowledgment of social entanglement is undeniably admirable, it has also written the permission slip for technology developers to think of themselves as the enforcers of medical prescription. There are few papers in this subfield that do not take "behavior change" as their object of study and design. One does not describe the actions of others as a "behavior" unless one deems their worth questionable. One also does not couple the word "change" with "behavior" so readily unless one believes it is individuals, and not institutions or political economies, that need changing.

I realize that I am now using ungenerous language, speaking more as the critic-partisan than the convener of arenas. Culture makes hypocrites of us all, and it is true that I find it difficult to summon affection for this sort of software, or to work with developers who are disinclined to acknowledge the political causes and consequences about which I care a great deal. In fact, there is more diversity and controversy within computer science than I am letting on. For example, Purpura et al. (2011) is a computer science paper in which the authors built a fictional weight loss encouragement system, "Fit4Life," by taking principles of persuasive computing to their logical extreme. It is a deliberate comment, in design form, on how easily unrestrained persuasive computing could spiral out of control. For example, Purpura and colleagues load up their system with multiple sensors used to "tunnel" users, guiding them through a staged set of interactions that communicate what to do next based on the sensors' data. They designed in alerts encouraging other users to shame someone who no longer wears the technology. Notably, the authors found that their audience could not distinguish earnest design from provocation.[8]

With that in mind, there is one last partisan point to be made. Whether the IT industry's acceptance of biomedical frameworks and cultural ideals about fit bodies happened through the trope of persuasive computing, or via more complicated routes, it has nevertheless resulted in an immunity to the basic facts of marketplace failure. Sixty percent of health-related apps fall into disuse after six months of ownership (Economist Intelligence Unit and Price Waterhouse Cooper 2012). The trade press considers such early abandonment to be a constraint on market growth (Rank 2014) because this figure suggests a lack of engagement and costly customer churn, not the effects of planned obsolescence. The problems of modern living these apps and devices were designed to solve (obesity and its various cousins) are problems that require much longer than six months to correct. This suggests that people are not using these products as intended, yet if anything, the industry has doubled down on gamification and images of strong, disciplined, lycra-ed bodies to articulate the value their products offer. When the private sector has not responded to market signals, we have perhaps the surest sign that a cultural logic more powerful than capitalism is at work.

## Time and Partial Indication

Biosensing systems have two fundamental things in common: the centrality of time, and a problematic relationship to indexicality. Tom Boellstorff (2013) reminds us that the words "data" and "dated" are etymologically related for a reason. Data always have a date—they are that which is stamped by time, recorded as having taken place. Data generated by these technologies may or may not be associated with a location, but it most certainly will be associated with a time, often called a "time stamp." This makes biosensor data largely time-series data.[9] This is no mere technical detail. As Sherman (chapter 2) observes, time is what makes it possible to treat data abstractly, and to create new abstractions from it. Data can only become meaningful when it is brought into relation to other data (Gitelman 2013; boyd and Crawford 2011), and time is the hinge that makes this possible both mathematically and socially. Mathematically speaking, when two time series co-vary, they co-vary across time, as in the correlation that says, "when my steps increase, so does my heart rate." Jumping from a single person to a population requires a decision about how time is to be handled. The correlation that says "people who take many steps also have high heart rates" contains no notion of time, and can be made by averaging all the data in each time series before correlating across a population. However, the second correlation does not follow from the first. We might imagine that people who take many steps have lower heart rates overall because exercise tends to lower resting heart rates while temporarily raising heart rate during exercise. If we reintroduce time through more sophisticated statistical techniques, however, a researcher can detect this more fine-grained pattern.

The ability to look for patterns in time, rather than just across a population, comes from the technological conditions which make it possible to sample things at much higher rates than a survey or health record data can. In a sense, sensors lay tracks in time (Day and Lury, chapter 3). The exact cadence of these tracks, or traces, depends on the sampling rate the sensor is set to, which can be anywhere from a second-by-second data collection, to once a day, to "when someone feels like it" in the case of manually initiated data collection. Where there are differences in sample rates, the calculation techniques can become complex, as the people processing the data must make a claim that variable X spiked at the "same time" as variable Y for practical purposes, even if their time stamps are not exactly the same. Similarly, where data have been collected from two different devices, if those devices do not use the same technique to record which time zone the person is in, chaos can ensue. A covariance in time is much harder to generate if one device/service adjusts how it records time when a person travels, and the other does not. Without good metadata, one can only guess which "5pm" those steps took place in.

Not only does time make data relate to other data, it also makes data relate to people, and to the broader cultural imaginations they possess. For example, where there is a spike in steps or heart rate, a sensor user might simply recall what else was happening when that spike occurred. In this way, the experiential qualities of time can be a more powerful analytical tool than mathematical correlation (Ruckenstein 2014). Similarly, data examined in the moment of, say, a bike ride, is experienced very differently than data designed to be contemplated post hoc. Aasarød (2012) describes the bodily sensations people have when they use continuous glucose monitors. Some use the devices to calibrate their own experiences of their body, to "learn" what a high or low level of glucose feels like by looking at it at the moment of physical sensation. Others effectively outsource that sensing to the device, which effectively tells them what to feel. Nevertheless, for both kinds of people it is *the moment of looking* that makes the tie between body and number possible.

In other contexts, longer time cycles are at stake. In Böhlen's work (chapter 10), water quality needed to be tracked over the course of a year, not just in the moment, to check that it was safe. The seasons had an effect on the water's physical attributes and therefore on the social practices around collecting and purifying it. Similarly, bodies themselves have temporal cycles, and need time to respond to new treatment regimes devised on the basis of biosensor data (see Kragh-Furbo et al., chapter 1). Institutions also have their temporal cycles. Changing biosensing practices can require carefully timed orchestration of both technology and policy (Gregory and Bowker, chapter 12). The pace at which institutional decisions are made can sometimes be disastrously out of sync with the rate of data collection (Böhlen, chapter 10). Could rapid sampling rates constitute a new round of space-time compression (Harvey 1989), quickening the pace of life? Perhaps, though data in the *longue durée* also matter (see Wolf, chapter 4), and there is no such thing as "real time" *per se*. How quick is "real"? Down to the hour? Minute? Nanosecond? What we can say for now is that biosensors mediate temporal calibrations among people, materials, and institutional processes.

Biosensing practices also share a difficult relationship to indexical forms of meaning making. Sensors are designed to indicate. They are designed to point to a phenomenon as if data were like smoke to a fire—that is, an index in a straightforwardly Peircian way. In practice, indications are hardly straightforward or clear. A single sensor can indicate many things. For example, activity monitors often use accelerometers to detect both steps taken and sleep quality, while elevated body temperature can indicate anything from ovulation to stress to influenza to Ebola. A raised heart rate might indicate stress, but is it stress the body experiences through exercise, known to reduce "stress" in a different sense? And what exactly does one look for in this heart rate—sustained elevation or spikes? A continuous sampling of heart rate as opposed to a pulse taken once a year in a doctor's office could indicate something entirely novel, and put someone down a very different path just by increasing the sampling rate. The human lifeworld that exists around a thing we might call "stress" is only partially evoked by what might be mechanically sensed. Conversely, what is mechanically sensed might not speak to "stress" at all but something entirely different (Leahu and Sengers 2014). In these ways, sensors point to a possible wider phenomenon, a whole, but do not make the exact contents of that whole evident (Nafus 2014). The problem is not that lay people are confused or lack expertise to make sense of sensor data; it is that the technology is itself confusing. For example, brain-imaging technology (PET scans) poses to neuroscientists exactly this kind of confusion around parts and wholes (Dumit 2004). Simple changes of color contrast in the PET image can produce wildly different interpretations of the underlying data.

The cultures that would connect lifeworlds and machineworlds are so nascent and diverse that those who endeavor to puzzle these issues through have much work ahead of them (Kragh-Furbo et al., chapter 1; Böhlen, chapter 10; Gregory and Bowker, chapter 12; Nafus 2014). To use Kragh-Furbo et al.'s phrase, data are overloaded with potential, and without further work, they remain mere potential. Taylor (chapter 11) calls our attention to the additional work necessary to make data culturally and socially meaningful, beyond the scientific work that would, say, establish the relationship between genotype and the physical expression of those genes. On the one hand, he points out that there are cultural, aesthetic, and social questions that go unasked of datasets, and argues that data collection and calculation are done in highly conservative—dare I say it, boring—ways. On the other hand, Estrin and De Paula Hanika (chapter 9) point to the rapid expansion in medical comprehension of sensor data for clinical intervention, hardly tedious. What these two contributions share is a notion that data can, in fact, be designed. A greater sense of intentionality in what data *should* be collected and calculated is likely to yield more productive sensing practices than treating datasets as stockpiles of found objects that inadvertently exude meaning.

## How This Book Is Organized

This book is organized to reflect where the conversations about biosensing actually are, not what kinds of conversation will prove satisfying in any one of those quarters. The various contributions to this book necessarily contain large differences among intellectual traditions, and differences in practical versus theoretical orientations. The authors are not all participating in exactly the same conversation, and neither is the public. My hope is that this collection can thicken some of these connections.

Leaving academia has only strengthened my belief that some academic concepts are too valuable to be left as matters of insider discussion. At the same time, it is foolish to pretend research is not research. In a research publication, there is no avoiding terms of art when they are useful, and simplifying a complex world is not the same thing as actually understanding it.[10] I have tried to find a way to expand engagement with public concerns, while still directly conveying the research, by asking three people doing important work outside the academy (Estrin, Wolf, and Mehta) to join the conversation happening in this small arena of ours.[11] Two of these chapters engage the scholarship directly, and offer their own thoughts in return. Estrin's offers an explanation of why she builds technologies in a particular way—important explanations that could go missing if buried under a wider social scientific argument. This was a genuine experiment, in as much as I wanted to know which ideas from the scholarly chapters these contributors would find interesting, and what other ideas they would want to raise for a largely social scientific audience.

In some senses, this editorial choice follows the longstanding tradition in anthropology of directly including voices of the people we study (Clifford and Marcus 1986). As anthropology no longer confines itself to studying the marginalized, we can no longer presume that it is the anthropologist's voice that is the voice of privilege. This is not a book written from the margins of social life, though I look forward to someone writing one with respect to biosensing. Here, including people who build technologies and communities does a different kind of work. It experiments with what kinds of conversations in the "center" could become possible if more voices from the "margins" of the social sciences and humanities were taken seriously. Being taken seriously is not the same thing as being agreed with, of course, or even sharing the same epistemological frame. However, these contributions give us grounds to ask practical questions about what it might look like for social scientists to intervene more directly in the trajectories that biosensors take.

Part I, "Biosensing and Representation," examines how data, personhood, and abstraction relate to one another. Mette Kragh-Furbo, Adrian Mackenzie, Maggie Mort, and Celia Roberts begin chapter 1 with perhaps the most urgent political question: *Do biosensors biomedicalize?* Using the case of direct-to-consumer genomics, they answer affirmatively, while also observing other social practices that cannot be accounted for by the biomedicalization thesis alone. They see new sites of "negotiation, contestation, and diversity that may not be fully biomedicalizable." Part of what makes room for diversity is the complexity of the datasets themselves. Layers upon layers of abstraction make the connection between DNA data and body not just partial but circuitous, far more indirect that the indexicality I described earlier. This creates room for, say, care and affection between people trying to make sense of the data, or attention to individual biography and experience. It also creates room for false hope. To work on this sort of data presupposes it could contain an answer to one's problems, when in fact there may not be an answer.

In chapter 2, Jamie Sherman takes an entirely different approach to the question of what data's abstractions do for people, and to people. The data that her research participants use are not as complex as in the first chapter, but this brings into sharper relief their connection to aesthetic practice, as opposed to technoscientific logics. Using the work of Walter Benjamin, she argues that we can think about data as a cultural medium of recording analogous to film and photography that came before it. Self-tracking data keep a quasi-abstracted account of one's activities, allowing the tracker to conduct tricks of proximity and distance. Much like the photographic practices of Benjamin's day, these maneuvers afford different vantage points from which to see and experience the self. This self-in-data is never the "whole self" but is comprised of details made separable by the technologies of the day.

In chapter 3, Sophie Day and Celia Lury argue that data cultures push on ideologies of the self more radically than in Sherman's account. They argue that contemporary cultures of observation expose the fictions we in the West tell ourselves about personhood—in other words, that there is such thing as an individual with clear boundaries, such that we can then also sensibly draw fixed rings around what is public and what is private. Instead, they argue that what we are really doing in acts of tracking is recursively producing those notions of private and public, individual and others, more or less on the fly. Their notion of the "dividual," drawn from the Melanesian ethnography of Marilyn Strathern, entails a personhood that is partible, constitutive of the relations it forges. It does not carry around an essential "core" that moves unchanged from one social relation to the next, as we like to tell ourselves. The dividual bears an uncanny relation to the personhood Sherman describes, which comes into being through attention to separable details. It is also not dissimilar from the "pixelated person" described by Greenfield in chapter 7. Could it be that pixelation becomes the technoscientific idiom with which the West tiptoes up to a notion of "dividuality," without, perhaps, fully embracing its ramifications in the way the Melanesians do?

Journalist and Quantified Self community founder Gary Wolf responds in chapter 4 to the material in part 1 with an observation about self-tracking enthusiasts: "These maneuvers of self-separation, carried out with varying degree of expertise, are unhesitatingly presented as techniques of enlightenment. Hasn't anybody noticed the trouble the self is in?" Perhaps not, even though anthropologists are quick to point it out. Wolf offers yet another way of thinking about self-tracking, by reminding us that most community members are also technology producers. In that industry, talk is relentlessly about the future. By comparison, putting digital breadcrumbs in the past by recording it numerically provides a rare opportunity for grounding in the here and now.

Part II, "Institutional Arrangements," focuses on the institutions of law, commerce, and medicine as they both shape and are shaped by biosensors. In Chapter 5, legal scholars Helen Nissenbaum and Heather Patterson also reject the notion of privacy as somehow fixed, but they do so for very different reasons than Day and Lury. They argue that privacy violations are experienced when there is a disruption in the expected flow of information. It is not that specific data types are inherently "sensitive," nor does the specific institutional context alone make data "private." For example, a blood pressure measurement collected in a clinical setting falls under U.S. medical privacy law (HIPAA), but that same data collected in a home by a consumer-grade device may not. If employees are going to be coerced into giving their employer or health insurance company blood pressure data, it matters little where or how the data were generated, or the nature of the data per se, because overriding this is a normative expectation that employers do not concern themselves with employees' bodies. These authors provide specific, practical guidance for how to trace where data flow, and how to surface the gap between expectations and reality in order to help designers and policymakers identify sources of privacy violation.

In chapter 6, Brittany Fiore-Gartland and Gina Neff help us understand how business school conceptualizations of markets are being mobilized to secure a place for biosensor companies within the U.S. health-care system. They point out that companies take aim at "disrupting" traditional medicine through biosensing by claiming to "cut out a middleman, while integrating seamlessly all the parts of the middleman's very system that will soon be made obsolete." They argue that companies skirt regulation by delivering "raw data" on an informational basis, yet deliver those data alongside encouragements to talk with a medical professional about it. This effectively outsources much of the interpretive work back to the medical system, without the firm having to pay for that work. The authors see the "democratization" talk used to legitimate such "disruption" as a kind of bait and switch. It mobilizes the sometimes-strong desires of patients for health systems to "give me my DAM data [i.e., data about me]," but ensures more control over the medical system for the "disrupting" firm than for individuals.

Dana Greenfield writes as both an anthropologist and medical professional. In chapter 7, she addresses the relationship between medicine and self-tracking. While Fiore-Gartland and Neff direct our attention toward a power struggle within a political economy, Greenfield directs our attention to the multiplicity of coexisting medical and paraclinical practices. She focuses on the "n of 1," a trope used within the Quantified Self community to talk about the relation between self-tracking and medical research. When we look at how "n of 1" is invoked, we find a polyvocal concept. Sometimes "n of 1" is about the open-ended tinkering with the protocols of care, which fits well with Mol's (2008) logic of care. It can also be a way to think about massive datasets that scale up to population levels and back down again to an individual, who would receive personalized treatments calculated through the difference between her and the population-level aggregation. It can yet again be a way to interject narrative form back into medical practice. Put together, though, the "n of 1" suggests that self-tracking can be usefully thought of as a paraclinical practice: "By taking up the tools of medicine, but not its claims to expertise, this is medicine turned inside out."

Rajiv Mehta is a Silicon Valley entrepreneur who reflects on the material in part II as someone who has had to make practical decisions about privacy by design and his relationship to the health-care system. In chapter 8, he helpfully observes that there are serious tradeoffs between preserving privacy by designing better user controls, and enacting legislation that targets harmful use of data (an example of similar policy in the UK can be found in chapter 3). Mehta also calls into question whether "disruption" is actually at work in this market. The apps he designed and sold are calendaring programs adapted for caregivers, and did not remotely come close to "skirting medical jurisdiction." Still, he had to contend with a powerful assumption that "health-related" meant the same thing as medicine, and at every turn was questioned about the extent to which his calendars had been medically vetted. This is not the way disruption works as traditionally understood. The aggressive treatment he received, simply for not giving biomedicine totalizing authority, suggests that more is going on here.

There are some things that only become clear by doing, rather than by commenting on the results of what was done. The final part III, "Seeing Like a Builder," offers an engineer's-eye view from the trenches of building technical systems. Here I have reversed the pattern of social scientific commentary followed by a response, and instead begin with an interview[12] with Deborah Estrin, a founder of Open mHealth. I asked Estrin to help us understand what it takes to move data between institutions. The hard part, she observes, is ensuring that data remain intelligible as they move from one party to the next. There is a tension here between Patterson and Nissenbaum's concern about privacy violations enabled by the free flow of data, and Estrin's concern about the careful technical decisions that need to be made to build systems that make "flows" possible at all. The tension is not over whether there are too few or too many controls on where data are exchanged. All of the authors agree on the importance of controls. Instead, the work of Open mHealth suggests a broader conceptual point. Universal free flow of data does not exist in the way that social science's extensive reliance on the term would have it. The trope of data "flowing" reflects our ability to imagine the connective qualities of data. It is easy to imagine how a piece of location data combined with heart rate data combined with yet more data can paint a detailed picture (and the truly frightening things that can happen when this picture is painted without our consent). However, the material realities do not come together as easily. Remember my earlier example of two services that do not handle time zones in the same way. The data cannot just "flow" between those services, even if the connecting pipes are there. There is friction (Edwards et al. 2011) between the datasets themselves, and nontrivial resources are required to remove that friction if someone is going to successfully paint a picture with it. With NSA-sized budgets, such friction is easily overcome, but not so for smaller firms and research projects. Just as there are services that happily expose data to the highest bidder, these frictions create points of nonexchange that hinder entirely appropriate medical research, clinical practice, and personal self-tracking.

In chapter 10, Marc Böhlen gives us a ringside seat to the tradeoffs and uncertainties of building biosensor systems. Böhlen reshapes the capacities of technical systems in an ongoing way, in response to the relationships he builds to both individuals and institutions. He reflects on a moment of calibrating water-testing equipment in Indonesia, in which the calibration of his technical system was really a kind of social and political calibration that made the Indonesian state more at ease with his presence. Through his actions, Böhlen makes evident the sheer complexity of maintaining multiple layers of socio-technical calibrations. Like Open mHealth, his data "flows" were a hard-won outcome of social and technical work. His shuttling between two social institutions, one state-based and focused on health, and the other a less formal but very powerful network of neighborhood organizations, also serves as an important reminder that the institutions that shape medicine and health do not necessarily fight for control over the domain in the way that Mehta experienced in the United States.

In chapter 11, Alex Taylor raises the question of what alternative forms of data might look like, by attempting to make different "cuts" of data. He takes to task the claims of big data proponents who argue that the promise of big data is to learn something new, of human value. If this is so, why do these same proponents launch so few challenges to the preexisting social categories that shape what is measured and where the data are stored? Taylor argues that there is room to do better if we take the stated promise at its word. He embarks on a small data collection project to point toward what goes unnarrated in commercial and civic systems, such as heart-rate monitors or bicycle-sharing programs. He shows the importance of datasets that do not fit the flat just-so stories of TED talks and marketing pitches. Taylor sums up the spirit of this collection when he says: "The computational substrates that ... are constitutive of big data should be given over to enlivening the relations, not flattening them. The trick here, as I see it, is to build in computational capacities that keep the vastness open, that don't slip too soon into neat classes—regimes even—of data that we know too well."

In the final chapter, Judith Gregory and Geoffrey C. Bowker further elaborate on what it might mean to keep the vastness open. By examining both microbiomes and genomes, their concept of the "data citizen" expands into the ecological. When they look at data they take the relationships, not the categories they supposedly refer to, to be ontologically prior. This opens up new spaces for design, and a much wider, and more inclusive, sense of who ought to be doing the designing. Such spaces include the design of policy, as well as objects. Indeed we could infer from their attention to aesthetic considerations that a more expanded space for design might also include rhetorical form alongside functional concerns.

## Notes

1. Readers curious about this sometimes vexed, sometimes productive form of public engagement might explore www.epicpeople.org and Denny and Sunderland (2014).

2. See Guthman (2011) for a critical take on the social dynamics that have led to constructing America's growing waistline as a medical problem.

3. Research from chapters 1, 3, 6, and 10 was supported through this program. Researchers were in no way restricted in whether, how, or when they could publish their results.

4. At the time of writing, nearly every Quantified Self group in a large city has a resident ethnographer. Early works include Watson (2013), Lupton (2014a), Dow Schüll (forthcoming), Boesel (2013), Williams (2013), and Nafus and Sherman (2014).

5. Boesel (2013) usefully distinguishes "lowercase qs" (the generic description for self-tracking practices) from "uppercase QS" (for Quantified Self, the group of enthusiasts who meet on a regular basis, and describe themselves as a lead user community).

6. Lupton's self-tracking "types" (2014b) make helpful progress here, in that they make explicit the relations between selves and others, but still put selves at the center. My desire is not to suggest these types are not useful—hardly—but to explore what happens if we can decenter selves entirely so as to revisit them anew.

7. Americangut.org.

8. Shteyngart's (2011) fictional satire of a biosensor-rich world captures the at-once toxic and comical social arrangements that are a natural extension of a gamified, biomedicalized world.

9. A notable exception to this rule is genome data, which technically speaking will contain a time stamp (the time at which the sample was taken or processed), but further sampling is largely meaningless.

10. It is a cruel irony that those who are most confused about the public value of the social sciences and humanities are among the quickest to demand simplistic explanations of what researchers do. This is a trap. Time, resources, and generous listening are required to get public and yes, economic, value out of research. If policymakers have trouble seeing the connection between social science and the matters of public import, they would do better to examine the absence of resources available to make this translation, and not the nature of the research itself.

11. Estrin is a computer scientist at Cornell University, but she speaks here as a founder of a nonprofit organization.

12. The interview format is something of a conceit. It indeed took place, though Estrin and her colleague Anna de Paula Hanika edited the text printed here.

## References

Aasarød, Askild Matre. 2012. "A Dislocated Gut Feeling: An Analysis of Cyborg Relations in Diabetes Self-Care." MA thesis, Aarhus University. Aarhus, Denmark.

ABI. 2014. "Ninety Million Wearable Computing Devices Will Be Shipped in 2014 Driven by Sports, Health, and Fitness." https://www.abiresearch.com/press/ninety-million-wearable-computing-devices-will-be-. Accessed 11/15/2014.

Boellstorff, Tom. 2013. "Making Big Data, in Theory." *First Monday* 18 (10). http://firstmonday.org/ojs/index.php/fm/article/view/4869. Accessed 11/15/2014.

Boesel, Whitney. 2013. "What Is the Quantified Self Now?" May 22. http://thesocietypages.org/cyborgology/2013/05/22/what-is-the-quantified-self-now/. Accessed 11/15/2014.

boyd, danah, and Kate Crawford. 2011. Six Provocations for Big Data. SSRN Scholarly Paper ID 1926431. Social Science Research Network, Rochester, NY; http://papers.ssrn.com/abstract=1926431. Accessed 11/15/2014.

Clifford, James, and George E. Marcus. 1986. *Writing Culture: The Poetics and Politics of Ethnography: A School of American Research Advanced Seminar*. Berkeley, CA: University of California Press.

Denny, Rita M., and Patricia L. Sunderland, eds. 2014. *Handbook of Anthropology in Business*. Walnut Creek, CA: Left Coast Press.

van Dijck, Jose. 2014. "Datafication, Dataism and Dataveillance: Big Data between Scientific Paradigm and Ideology." *Surveillance & Society* 12 (2): 197–208.

Dow Schüll, Natasha. Forthcoming. *Keeping Track: Personal Informatics, Self-Regulation, and the Data-Driven Life*. New York: Farrar, Straus, and Giroux.

Dumit, J. 2004. *Picturing Personhood: Brain Scans and Biomedical Identity*. Princeton, NJ: Princeton Univ Press.

Economist Intelligence Unit and Price Waterhouse Cooper. 2012. "Emerging mHealth: Paths for Growth." http://www.managementthinking.eiu.com/sites/default/files/downloads/Emerging%20mHealth.pdf.

Edwards, Paul, Matthew Mayernik, Archer Batcheller, Geoffrey Bowker, and Christine Borgman. 2011. "Science Friction: Data, Metadata, and Collaboration." *Social Studies of Science* 41 (5): 667–690.

Fogg, B. J. 2002. "Persuasive Technology: Using Computers to Change What We Think and Do." *Ubiquity* (December) (5): 89–120.

Gitelman, Lisa, ed. 2013. *"Raw Data" Is an Oxymoron*. Cambridge, MA: The MIT Press.

Guthman, Julie. 2011. *Weighing In: Obesity, Food Justice, and the Limits of Capitalism*. 1st ed. Berkeley: University of California Press.

Harvey, David. 1989. *The Condition of Postmodernity*. Vol. 14. Oxford: Blackwell.

Latour, Bruno. 2004. "Why Has Critique Run out of Steam? From Matters of Fact to Matters of Concern." *Critical Inquiry* 30 (2): 225–248.

Leahu, Lucian, and Phoebe Sengers. 2014. "Freaky: Performing Hybrid Human-Machine Emotion." In *Proceedings of the 2014 Conference on Designing Interactive Systems*, 607–616. DIS '14. New York: ACM.

Lupton, Deborah. 2014a. "Self-Tracking Cultures: Towards a Sociology of Personal Informatics." In *Proceedings of the 26th Australian Computer—Human Interaction Conference on Designing Futures: The Future of Design*, 77–86. December 2–5. University of Technology, Sydney, Australia. New York: ACM.

Lupton, Deborah. 2014b. "Self-Tracking Modes: Reflexive Self-Monitoring and Data Practices." SSRN Scholarly Paper ID 2483549. Rochester, NY: Social

Science Research Network; http://papers.ssrn.com/abstract=2483549. Accessed 11/14/2014.

Mol, Annemarie. 2008. *The Logic of Care: Health and the Problem of Patient Choice*. London: Routledge.

Mort, Maggie, Celia Roberts, and Blanca Callén. 2013. "Ageing with Telecare: Care or Coercion in Austerity?" *Sociology of Health & Illness* 35 (6): 799–812.

Mort, Maggie, Celia Roberts, Jeannette Pols, Miquel Domenech, Ingunn Moser, and The EFORTT investigators. 2013. "Ethical Implications of Home Telecare for Older People: A Framework Derived from a Multisited Participative Study." *Health Expectations*, 18: 438–449.

Nafus, Dawn. 2014. "Stuck Data, Dead Data, and Disloyal Data: The Stops and Starts in Making Numbers into Social Practices." *Distinktion: Scandinavian Journal of Social Theory* 15 (2): 208–222.

Nafus, Dawn, and Jamie Sherman. 2014. "This One Does Not Go Up to 11: The Quantified Self Movement as an Alternative Big Data Practice." *International Journal of Communication* 8 (11): 1784–1794.

Neff, Gina. 2013. "Why Big Data Won't Cure Us." *Big Data* 1 (3): 117–123.

November, Joseph. 2012. *Biomedical Computing: Digitizing Life in the United States*. Baltimore: The Johns Hopkins University Press.

Pols, Jeannette. 2011. "Wonderful Webcams: About Active Gazes and Invisible Technologies." *Science, Technology & Human Values*, 36 (4): 451–473.

Purpura, Stephen, Victoria Schwanda, Kaiton Williams, William Stubler, and Phoebe Sengers. 2011. "Fit4Life: The Design of a Persuasive Technology Promoting Healthy Behavior and Ideal Weight." In *Proceedings of the SIGCHI Conference on Human Factors in Computing Systems*, 423–432. CHI '11. New York: ACM.

Rank, Judith. 2014. "Platform Wars for the Quantified Self." October 20. http://research.gigaom.com/report/platform-wars-for-the-quantified-self/. Accessed November 15, 2014.

Ruckenstein, Minna. 2014. "Visualized and Interacted Life: Personal Analytics and Engagements with Data Doubles." *Societies* (Basel, Switzerland) 4 (1): 68–84.

Shteyngart, Gary. 2011. *Super Sad True Love Story: A Novel*. New York: Random House Trade Paperbacks.

Strathern, Marilyn. 2001. Virtual Society? Get Real! Abstraction and Decontextualisation: An Anthropological Comment or: E for Ethnography." *Cambridge Anthropology* 22 (1): 52–66.

Till, Chris. 2014. "Exercise as Labour: Quantified Self and the Transformation of Exercise into Labour." *Societies* (Basel, Switzerland) 4 (3): 446–462.

Watson, S. 2013. "Living with Data: Personal Uses of the Quantified Self." MPhil thesis, University of Oxford.

Weiser, Mark. 1991. "The Computer for the 21st Century." *Scientific American* 265 (3): 94–104.

Whitson, Jennifer R. 2013. "Gaming the Quantified Self." *Surveillance & Society* 11 (1/2): 163–176.

Williams, Kaiton. 2013. "The Weight of Things Lost." In *Proceedings of CHI '13*. April 27–May 2. Paris, France. New York: ACM. http://www.personalinformatics.org/docs/chi2013/williams.pdf. Accessed August 15, 2015.

# I

# Biosensing and Representation

Part I considers the cultures of representation in biosensing practices. Biosensors, like other sensors, are designed to create a trace back to the physical world in some way. They contain built-in assumptions about what their users are supposed to see, by calling attention to some things at the expense of other things. Biosensors, and sensors more generally, can sometimes make it seem as if the things that cannot be sensed electronically might as well exist beyond the edge of a cliff. In this way, biosensors propose a "hypothesis of sight," as Day and Lury suggest, following the artist Mel Bochner. That is, they propose a boundary concerning what is supposed to be visible and what is not. However, they are also used in cultural contexts that have their own cultures of observation, and understandings about how representation is supposed to be done. Sometimes these cultural contexts are part and parcel of the very same labs in which biosensors are developed, while at other times these contexts can be squarely located in artistic practice, biography making, or everyday life.

In a sense, we have been here before. Many scholars will remember the early days of Internet studies, when the Internet was imagined be its own "space" or "world." To break the imagined wall between "virtual" and "real" was to see what you were not supposed to, as if falling off the edge of the (virtual) world. For some observers, this mutable space was a liberating extension of self-representation, while others noted that social categories were hardly escaped in online practices. Still, we can plainly see a hypothesis of sight at work here. To propose that wires, modems and digital data constituted a "space" is to propose a theory of what one is meant to see and not see.

Unlike virtual worlds, biosensors ground their hypotheses of sight in very specific physical, often bodily, phenomena, and thus do not create spaces as such. Whereas in the early days of the Internet many researchers were struck by the mutability of digital forms, here it is the narrowness of digital readings that is so remarkable. A heart rate. A genome. A glucose level. It is this reduction that puts us on less steady ground, forcing a degree of uncertainty about what kind of picture is being painted with these already partial representations. Biosensor data are not more real, of course, just differently virtual. They do not represent identities and selves in exactly the same way as online avatars do, but they nevertheless irrefutably contain representations of people.

To render a person or a physical object into data is to take a partial representation, not a picture of the whole thing. That partial representation is further subdivided into parts that can be separated from one another. Each data point represents a person, or a thing, at a certain a point in time, which makes it separable from other data. The separability poses challenges for the ability to see the humanity at the other end. Divide and divide, it gets harder to detect the humanity within the data, and yet, like Camphor's dust, a silhouette of it remains.

Furthermore, those divided parts do not stand on their own—they must be reassembled to be useful. There are infinite choices to make about how to reassemble data: is it a pattern within one person, an average across many, or a wider claim of some kind? Perhaps, as in some wearable technologies, only some of the data are made available to the technology user while the full dataset is very much visible to the company. Whatever the reassembly strategy, bringing biosensor data back together into a kind of coherence introduces complexity and indirectness into whatever it is the data are meant to represent. In these ways, biosensors do not simplify our world, but instead propose a reductive hypothesis of sight. This ultimately makes things more complex, not less.

All four chapters in this section consider how these reductions and separations paradoxically generate more complex layers of meaning. Each author develops a different aspect of this theme. For example, Sherman notes that when images, text, or numbers are framed as data per se, they become part of a broader history of Western visual form that has always grappled with the losses involved in making copies, or taking only parts. To render a piece of text, or an image, or a number as data is to abstract it from the bodies, and the senses of self, from which it comes. This abstraction is also what makes things commensurable, even if they were not in their original forms. Commensurability, in a sense, is the power of biosensor data, and also their problem.

Similarly, Kragh-Furbo et al. observe the "relentlessly monotonous" character of genetic data—a description reminiscent of Walter Benjamin's concern about the "hellish repetition" of an earlier modernity. Four compounds, represented by four letters (ATGC), create rich combinations that in turn fill vast libraries of genomic sequences. This monotony, however relentless, enables a combinatorial logic. It also requires layers of mathematical forms far more complex than an average to cohere those combinations into a meaningful description of what DNA does. Between the combinations and layers of calculation, DNA sequences become less of a determinant than they might at first appear. The monotony is overwhelmed by variety and complexity. Because the data are separable from one another, and the bodies from which they come, categories can get unstable. When we say "genome" often we think of a genome referring to a person, or a species, but the same sequences can be separated from that organism and traced across multiple organisms. Stable referents cannot be assumed.

Day and Lury, in contrast, add a recursive logic to the layers produced by datafication. By looking at the wider cultures of observation in which biosensor data is situated, they find that Western notions of self and other, private and public, contain a recursive quality independent of the presence of data. When data that refer to self (and other) come into play, they follow the recursive pattern already in place through their own logic of looping back and laying traces. It is these traces where we start to get into trouble. To ask "What is my data as opposed to other people's data?" is to ask both about a trace—how the data got to where it did—and to ask about where self ends and other begins. Those things recurse, making it an impossible question to answer, but answer it we must. Claims about self and other underwrite ownership claims and claims that assert privacy rights. When we talk about privacy or ownership, we are rarely talking about privacy or ownership per se. We are really talking about social distance, about otherness, or about social systems we would rather not participate in, even if we participate anyway, unwillingly. The digital trace disallows the opportunity to erase the connections that are already there, but that we would prefer not to have.

Wolf closes part I by noting how data's reductions also serve a biographical purpose. In this sense, both Wolf's and Day and Lury's contributions develop notions of how data reshape the ongoing social construction of time and space. The people with whom Wolf primarily works live in Silicon Valley, a world as mutable and self-created as those in early descriptions of online life. The ability for data to ground a connection to the past matters when your social world is made up of meetings, TED videos, and talk of the future. In this sense, Wolf is inverting some of the logic that Sherman proposes. In Sherman's work, it is the original form—the form not yet made into data—that is on steadier ground, and in Wolf's, the nondata forms are anything but steady. Put together, though, we can see that both kinds of social logics could very well be in play, depending on the situation at hand.

# 1

# Do Biosensors Biomedicalize? Sites of Negotiation in DNA-Based Biosensing Data Practices

Mette Kragh-Furbo, Adrian Mackenzie, Maggie Mort, and Celia Roberts

> We see new forms of agency, empowerment, confusion, resistance, responsibility, docility, subjugation, citizenship, subjectivity, and morality. There are infinite new sites of negotiation, percolations of power, alleviations as well as instigations of suffering.
>
> A. E. Clarke et al. (2003, 185)

Do biosensors biomedicalize? If *biomedicalization* encompasses, as Clarke et al. (2003, 183) argued more than a decade ago, "the key processes occurring in the domains of health, illness, medicine and bodies especially but not only in the West," then we might expect health biosensors to exemplify the commercial, service-oriented, risk-focused, technoscientizing, knowledge-transforming, body- and identity-morphing processes of biomedicalization. As we will see in the case of DNA microarray-based biosensing, they may well biomedicalize. But DNA-based data also open onto potentially diverse and dense forms of biosensing practice. By virtue of its entanglements with medicine, digital media, pharmaceuticals, biotechnology, forensics, kinship, heredity, and genealogy, DNA is overloaded with biomedicalizing potential. At the same time, precisely because of this overloading of potential, and as DNA becomes a broader matter of biosensing, new sites appear of negotiation, percolation of power, and alleviation and instigation of suffering.

Although they are not typical biosensors, there is much to be learned about biosensing practice from how DNA microarray-based data circulate and percolate into spaces of risk, distribution of knowledge, and senses of health and illness. But in order to see this, we need to look away from the more highly publicized biomedical DNA-data events. The Human Genome Project and the patenting of the BRCA1 genes by the company Myriad Genetics are two high-profile examples of the politico-economic constitution of the "Biomedical TechnoService Complex, Inc." (Clarke et al. 2003) in which technoscientific innovations are corporatized and privatized. Similarly, on learning she had inherited a form of the BRCA1 gene associated with breast and ovarian cancer, Angelina Jolie criticized the costs of the tests for these genes (around $3,000) (Jolie 2013). Viewed in terms of these events, DNA-based biosensing fits easily within "biomedicalization" (Clarke et al. 2003) in which biomedicine is said to have reorganized from *the inside out* to become technoscientific. This means that technical, informational, organizational, and institutional infrastructures are remade via the creation of new social forms and practice that transform knowledge production, distribution, information management, and consumption.

At the same time, for over a decade, DNA microarrays of increasing density and sophistication have become sensing devices in a wide variety of research applications, mostly *outside* clinical settings. Data produced using microarrays in these settings depend heavily on a vast accumulation of DNA-related biological data. On this somewhat yet-to-be-validated research front, DNA-based biosensing points toward an open and expanding horizon. DNA microarray tests for inherited disease are not as accurate as the specific genetic tests Angelina Jolie refers to,[1] but they are significantly cheaper, and they test for many hundreds of possible risks, propensities, and susceptibilities. The current cost for the most widely known microarray-based tests offered by the well-known direct-to-consumer DNA testing company 23andMe, Inc. is $99. There is a certain "disintermediation" associated with these tests that biomedicalization does not describe so well. The use of DNA microarrays in genetic testing is no longer practiced solely within the clinic and academic laboratory, but travels widely across digital and commercial spheres and as a biosensing practice taken up locally and (re)interpreted by diverse social groups and individuals. An example is the online platform openSNP (www.opensnp.org), a nonprofit that enables people to openly share their genetic data with interested researchers and others; there are also many online support groups where people discuss and negotiate the meaning of their genetic data for genealogical purposes as well as in relation to a variety of health concerns. The way these data are taken up might be seen as engendering social spaces in which power-laden practices of knowing, prediction, making promises, sensing, and caring might be negotiated differently. We explore one such social space in the second part of the chapter, but first, we introduce the microarray as a biosensor and its highly leveraged and derivative data. Important to note is that its technical specificities cannot be brushed aside as mere technical details, but they indeed form part of the rich data ecology of DNA-based biosensing.

## Microarrays as Biosensors

Physically, as their name suggests, microarrays are small square devices, not much larger than a matchbox, and roughly the same thickness as a typical computer chip. Their miniature size and the fact that they routinely generate large amounts of digital data, derived from photo-optronic scanning[2] of the millions of wells on the microarrays, fits the general idea of a contemporary biosensor. DNA microarrays are sometimes called "labs-on-a-chip" or "micro total analysis systems." While we focus almost exclusively on human DNA in this chapter, DNA microarrays have been designed for a wide variety of settings ranging from environmental monitoring to infectious disease monitoring (Chua et al. 2011; Thiruppathiraja et al. 2011). In general, biosensors contain some biologically reactive element along with transducers[3] and inscriptive mechanisms (Banica 2012). DNA microarrays are not elementary textbook biosensors. In a typical biosensor, a biologically sensitive element is connected to a signal output or display via some kind of electrical interface (e.g., electrodes that measure a change in charge). Although they resemble large-scale integrated circuits, DNA microarrays are not electronic or electrochemical. They do contain biologically reactive chains of DNA molecules, but they lack the transducers that connect biological/biochemical activity of DNA to an electrical signal or to digital data. For microarrays, the transduction between biological activity and digital data occurs in a microarray scanner, which is a substantial benchtop laboratory instrument, sometimes highly automated with laboratory robots handling thousands of arrays per day. In the microarray scanner, lasers and digital optics convert fluorescing traces of biological reactivity of DNA into digital data. Figure 1.1 contains an example.

The "genetic tests"—although that is an overly broad term for what is more specifically "SNP-based genotyping of individuals"—we focus on here depend on several hundred thousand DNA fragments arrayed on the microarrays. While microarrays can be made to order for specific purposes by commercial producers or in well-equipped research facilities, standard microarrays are widely available for research into human biology and disease. The consumer genetic tests we are discussing here utilize off-the-shelf DNA microarrays from companies such as Affymetrix, Illumina, Agilent, Eppendorf, and Applied Microarrays; currently, 23andMe uses the Illumina iSelect custom chip (23andMe 2013).

DNA microarrays were originally developed for gene expression profiling in 1995 (Schena et al. 1995). In a typical microarray-based

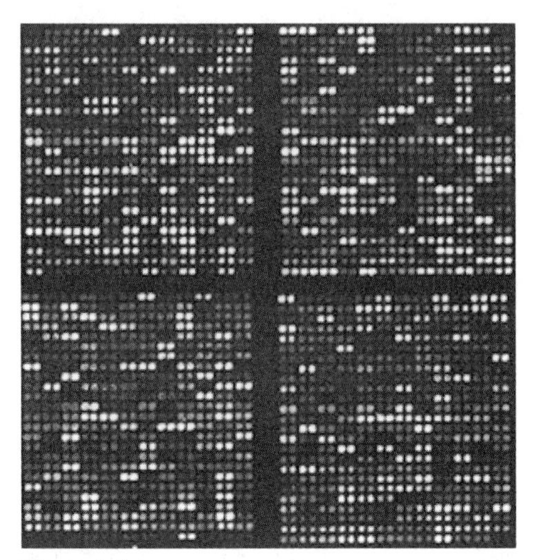

**Figure 1.1**
DNA microarray. Source: NASA, Creative Commons Public Domain.

experiment or test, a dissolved sample of DNA obtained from a patient or client flows across the microarray glass slide. Relatively quickly, fragments of DNA in the fluid sample bind with DNA fragments that are fixed on the array if they are complementary to it. Photo-optronic sensors in a microarray scanner measure the amount of each of the DNA fragments. By careful choice of which fragments of DNA go on the array, researchers can measure many different biological processes. Microarrays are therefore used widely in recent life sciences, in microbial ecology, biomedical research, pathology, and public health settings. They have had less success in clinical settings due to problems of standardizing the analysis of the data they produce (Shi et al. 2010). They can be used to profile levels of gene expression, to identify organisms in samples, to study the epigenetic landscape of genomes (the way their shape changes in response to environmental events), and above all, for *genotyping*—characterizing an individual in terms of how they differ from a group or population of individuals.

DNA microarrays or "gene chips" complicate any biomedicalizing reading of them not so much by virtue of their physical form, but because their capacity to detect specific fragments of DNA in samples explosively expands the potential range of DNA-based biosensing. Since the molecular biology "revolution" of the 1970s and the subsequent genomic "revolution" of the 1990s (emblematized in the Human Genome Project),

DNA sequences have emerged as ubiquitous deep readouts of biological activity in almost every life science. Huge accumulations of DNA data began with the Human Genome Project and exponentially multiply today, for instance, in the 1000 Genomes project of 2007 (Siva 2008) and the ENCODE—Encyclopedia of DNA Elements (Encode Consortium 2012). A cantilevered architecture of cross-linked scientific databases numbering in hundreds—GenBank, Ensembl, dbGAP, Uniprot, dbSNP—has grown up around DNA, RNA, and protein (amino acid) sequence data. By virtue of their origin in publicly funded research, much of the data are readily accessible. The rich linkage and metadata of these databases means that any given DNA sequence of interest can be tracked, annotated, compared, and interpreted along a multitude of paths between organisms (human-mouse-rat-monkey-rabbit-e.coli-yeast-etc.), into biochemical and metabolic processes, or into ecological and geographical information about species and populations. Despite, or perhaps because of their relentlessly monotonous character—the letters GATC in endless varying sequences—DNA sequence data are probably the mostly richly layered and leveraged form of data in contemporary sciences (Stevens 2013). A typical genome browser (see the Genome Browser at UCSC[4]) exemplifies this layering and leveraging. It invites selection, comparison, and superimposition of various lines of sequence data.

The rich data ecology of DNA sequences animates and troubles, we suggest, the biomedicalizing potential of microarrays. On one hand, it is a nutrient-rich broth for analysis and interpretation of health and illness in molecular-digital terms; on the other hand, the microarray data, no matter how concretely *indexical* (in the Peircean sense of contiguously signifying something in its measurements) it may be, it is indelibly *derivative*. That is, like financial derivatives, its apparent referentiality to a state of affairs in the world—an inherited propensity, a bodily trait, an environmental event, a disease state—relies on the highly statistically and biologically leveraged value materialized in the DNA data ecologies. This opens up biosensing to forms of negotiation, contestation, and diversity that may not be fully biomedicalizable.

## Leveraged and Derivative Data

To illustrate something of the derivative and leveraged flow of microarray data, consider the major shifts in DNA microarray practice. During the first years of their appearance in the mid-1990s, microarrays were mainly used to measure levels of expressions of specific genes in organisms. As scientific understandings of genomes (the whole complement of DNA in an organism) and genes developed, so too did the realization that patterns of gene expression associated with variations were exceedingly complex (see Keller [2000]) for perhaps the standard account of this realization). Single genes only occasionally predict high risk of disease (the so-called Mendelian or heritable diseases are rare, although around 1,000 genes are known to be involved) or some trait such as eye color, capacity to metabolize alcohol, or height (Yang et al. 2010). Perhaps, then, complex interactions of gene variants (alleles) might be responsible? This intuition of complex patterns of interaction motivated attempts to map the variations in human genomes in much greater detail. Beginning in the 1990s and augmented greatly by microarray-based studies, minute DNA variations scattered across regions of the genome emerged as possible markers of an individual's inherited propensity to disease or other traits. These variations, while difficult to map in detail, could at least be labeled as SNPs (single nucleotide polymorphisms) or single nucleic acid mutations. For human genomes comprising around three billion DNA base pairs and less than twenty thousand genes, more than a million SNPs have been mapped. The key finding of all this mapping of minute variations has been this: individuals who display a particular SNP at one site often predictably carry specific SNPs at other nearby variant sites. This correlation between scattered SNPs is known as linkage disequilibrium. It has become the basis of the many so-called "Genome Wide Association Studies" that search for associations between inherited patterns of SNPs and disease/traits.

To add a further level of complexity, global research projects such as the Human Haplotype Mapping Project—HapMap (The International HapMap Consortium 2005)—explored population-wide patterns of variations, yielding a further wave of microarray datasets, this time describing in increasingly intricate and systematic detail the common variations across the genomes of several hundred humans chosen carefully from four populations (Han in Beijing, Yoruba in Ibadan, Japanese in Tokyo, Central European from Utah). With this map of variation between major populations in hand, as well as the thousands of studies that had identified associations between SNPs and diseases or traits (Burton et al. 2007), microarrays could be designed to detect SNPs for particular population groups. Contemporary commercial microchips, such as the Affymetrix Genome-Wide Human SNP Array 6.0, are able to test for close to one million SNPs and one million copy number variations (http://www.

affymetrix.com). The biosensor then embodies a configured knowledge of population variations.

We have said little yet about the ways in which microarray-based DNA detection for a given individual sample can be connected to these maps of the inherited patterns of variation associated with diseases and traits. Like the financial derivatives mentioned earlier, the associations between SNPs and disease/traits are highly numerically leveraged. That is, they stand on many crosshatched layers of data, inference, modeling, and testing. The statistical inferences on which the associations rely are highly sophisticated since a DNA microarray is effectively running thousands or millions of experiments in parallel. Such inferences rely on multi-faceted mathematical constructs generated through algorithmic processes that begin with the image analysis of the chip and range to detection of gene-gene interactions in complex but common diseases (arthritis, Alzheimer's, cancers, etc). We do not discuss these models in any depth here, but it is important to recognize that much sought-after associations between traits/diseases and patterns of SNPs have occasioned strenuous and ongoing statistical modeling efforts on the part of genomic researchers. The toolboxes of computer science and statistics have been effectively ransacked for pattern recognition, data mining, and machine learning techniques that can detect the associations between hundreds and thousands of SNPs: neural networks, random forests, penalized regression, ridge regression, AdaBoost, and support vector machines are just some of the techniques in use (Szymczak et al. 2009). Detection of gene interactions in SNP-based genome-wide association is not a solved problem, and genome-wide association studies of the heritability of traits have often been wildly speculative (see, for example, microarray-based studies of entrepreneurship [Groenen et al. 2008]).

All of this database and statistically leveraged complexity means that SNP-based genotyping data produced from DNA microarrays have no simple, direct indexical connection to living bodies. Although these tests are called "direct to consumer" because they do not pass through a clinic or biomedical expert's hands, they are anything but direct. At many points in the flow of data running between a microarray and a predicted association with disease or some other propensity, scientific knowledge, techniques, devices, platforms models, and inferences intervene. The knowledges, techniques, devices, models, and inferences must frequently themselves adjust in response to other developments in genomics (such as the advent of global population-variation mapping projects, and case control studies on increasingly large cohorts). The highly mediated paths running between a body and the results of an SNP-based genotyping test are susceptible to many divergences, and they attract expectations, promises, hopes, and other forms of potentialization that crisscross between commercial and scientific, biomedical and digital, research and everyday life.

## Genetic Data Outside the Clinic

Increasingly, SNP data themselves move outside the laboratory and the clinic. It has been well established that genetic information has a life outside the institutions of biomedicine. Arribas-Ayllon, Featherstone, and Atkinson (2011) for example, study the circulation of genetic risk information among individuals and families as "practical ethics." Marina Levina (2010) explores how sharing one's genetic data is an act of good citizenship and therefore good for the network society. Kate O'Riordan (2010) explores a variety of "genomic incorporations" in the contemporary media ecology including the digital mediations of the genome, and Alessandro Delfanti (2012) explores what he calls "garage biology" and the questions it raises about participation, expertise, open access, neoliberalism, and academic capitalism. What we understand by genetic data and their technologies and how we practice those is necessarily multiple. Anne Kerr (2004, 168) points to this when she writes: "Genetic knowledge and the research and technologies with which it is associated mean many things to different people. They can be both mundane and unusual, helpful and oppressive. In order to understand these rich and dynamic processes we must move beyond the narrow categories of patient or lay expert, to look at genetics in the wider context of people's lives." We leave aside therefore questions about the individual and clinical utility of DTC genetic testing (see e.g., McGuire and Burke 2008; Foster, Mulvihill, and Sharp 2009; Hauskeller 2011; Spencer and Lockwood 2011; Curnutte and Testa 2012; Groves and Tutton 2013) or the problems of whether or not people should have "direct" access to their genetic data (see e.g., ACMG 2008; EASAC 2012; Howard and Borry 2012). Rather we focus on the negotiations of DNA data that assemble multiple bodies, interactions, knowledges, and technologies outside or peripheral to the formalized interactions of markets and clinics. But how do genetic data matter outside these formal settings?

As a part of her doctoral research, Kragh-Furbo observed an online forum for people living with a chronic illness and followed conversations among a group of the forum members who discuss, question, negotiate, and carefully study DNA data, the scientific literature, wikis, methylation and detox reports, and forum threads and other websites in an attempt to "get a plan" and "truly understand" rather than merely speculate, on what is often described as the "path to healing." This kind of care-work occurs after direct-to-consumer genetic testing. Processes of care-work reconfigure genetic data as they move across and in between interfaces, hardware, and people's lives. The data circulate within a complex, multilayered problematization that accompanies the contested nature of a chronic illness and the lives of people with this illness. But for the purpose of this chapter, we focus on one specific practice that a group of people on an online forum has taken up in an effort to get better.

The subforum in question—we will call it "SNPNet"—is a mix of senior members, newcomers, and lurkers who attempt to improve their treatment protocols by connecting their genotyping results (in addition to other tests results) to knowledge of metabolic pathways. There are between fifteen and twenty active senior members posting on SNPNet and an unknown number of lurkers who occasionally appear on the site. The online space has within a few years become a kind of "knowledge hub," rich in personal (illness and treatment) narratives and lay expertise on the topics of SNPs and methylation deficiencies. Briefly, methylation is the process of donating methyl groups to molecules such as DNA. The methylation reactions are important to metabolism, for example the metabolism of nutrients from our diets. Members of SNPNet have in particular been supportive of Amy Yasko's work on methylation and autism. Yasko holds a PhD in microbiology and immunology from Albany Medical College, New York, and cofounded the biotech companies Biotix Inc. (with Arta Motadel) and Oligos Etc. Inc. (with Roderic Dale), but has since left to start the company Holistic Health International and her private alternative health-care practice. In her book *Pathways to Recovery*, she describes methylation deficiencies as the under- or overactivation of methylation, which is "a key cellular pathway that promotes detoxification, controls inflammation, and balances the neurotransmitters [and] can result in mood and emotional shifts as well as liver, pancreas, stomach, intestinal, adrenal, thyroid, and hormonal imbalances" (Yasko 2004, 15). Treatment protocols have been suggested to help optimize these methylation deficiencies and restore methylation function, and with the help of genetic testing, it is suggested that it is possible to target these biochemical imbalances with "the missing nutritional ingredients that the body cannot adequately produce itself due to genetic mutations" (ibid. 23).

The theory that you can treat and repair metabolic processes through nutritional support is not Amy Yasko's alone. Parents of and health-care practitioners working with children with autism began experimenting with high doses of B-vitamins during the 1960s, and to give one example, the Autism Research Institute, founded in 1967, experiments with nutritional supplements to treat mental and development disabilities and talks about an "emergent picture" of the "biochemistry of autism" (see Chloe Silverman's [2012] study of autism and biomedicine). However, these methods of treatment have been questioned. In an article on autism and the use of DNA testing to recommend alternative therapies, Janet Woodcock, the director of the Center for Drug Evaluation and Research at the American Food and Drug Administration (FDA), has been quoted as saying: "A lot of this skims on the edge of health fraud" (Langreth and Lauerman 2012). Others including members of SNPNet have also expressed concerns about Amy Yasko's scientific credentials as well as her motivation for helping patients and advancing her treatment protocol.

Yasko operates from her alternative health-care practice in Bethel, Maine, through her online discussion group and via her company Holistic Health International, which sells genetic tests and the supplements that are recommended on her treatment protocol. She has not gained approval from the FDA for any of her tests. But neither has 23andMe, which offers SNP-based genotyping that members on SNPNet regard as the "cheap" and do-it-yourself (DIY) alternative to Yasko's $495 DNA methylation pathway analysis. Yasko includes in her genetic test "an individualized protocol for health optimization" whereas people who have had their DNA genotyped by 23andMe have to work out a treatment plan for themselves. Although these are two separate genetic tests offered by two different companies—one testing for thirty-one SNPs, the other for approximately six hundred thousand SNPs—the two intertwine to form part of this genetic data practice in very specific ways.

**Learning to Sense**

On SNPNet, questions such as "What can I do to better understand my 23andMe data?," "What do I need to know?," and "How do I get started on this?" have often been asked. Such questions presume that something worthwhile can be gleaned from the data provided and that the members learn which available resources to access, how to use them, and how to talk about SNPs and methylation. This sense of prospect and potential is evident throughout the SNPNet discussion group and, in particular, there is a strong focus on learning how to realize the potential of direct-to-consumer genetic testing. In Jean Lave and Etienne Wenger's terms (Lave and Wenger 1991), this can be described as a form of learning through participation in a "community of practice" in which learning is a relational and distributed process and itself an improvised practice. SNPNet members continually negotiate the meaning of the genetic data, the methylation and detox reports, and the scientific literature, and come up with partial answers and plans that for a time will make sense until those are disrupted by new findings and experiences. In this sense, there is a constant movement between practices of reading and studying and the practice of eating, in which members become what one of them describes as their own "lab rats" in their experiments with nutritional supplements. Taking the supplements is private practice, but practice that is socially and materially organized.

A lot of work is required to make sense of genetic data, as many of the subforum members sometimes painfully come to realize, and as is implied by the foregoing discussion of the DNA data ecology and the derivative, statistically leveraged character of test results. Getting the genetic data is described as easy (if you can afford it, that is), but making sense of the data can in contrast be hard work, especially when you know little to nothing about human genetics and biochemistry.

Making sense of one's genetic data and biochemical pathways is a slow learning process that takes time, effort, and resources. It is described as opening an enormous Pandora's Box of new material that most likely will take months to understand. Yasko (2004, 6) also writes: "Even using all these resources [her book, website, and online discussion group], understanding the science will not happen overnight; it is a slow process as you immerse yourself." But there is hope, if you ask Yasko. Invest time (and money) in the program (Yasko's methylation protocol) and you'll be able "to take charge of your own health"—that is how it is imagined by Yasko. OnSNPNet, the sense is that there is "great potential in working this out" and yet so much to learn. The difference between Yasko's approach and what most SNPNet members are doing is that Yasko will be "teaching you about the processes going on in the body so that you are in a better position to make informed choices on the path to health and wellness." In contrast, SNPNet members will get involved in a kind of improvised learning, not to make an informed choice and achieve health and wellness, but to get some direction and advice on how to *just get better*.

Getting better takes practice. It is about reading up on genetics and methylation and learning what it all means, but also knowing which questions to ask. Slowly, SNPNet members learn how to participate in a genetic data practice that involves asking a lot of questions. Being curious and asking questions, one of them writes, is a crucial part of "what will get us out of this." But to be able to ask those important questions and become, as least, competent *enough* to participate to some extent in this genetic data practice, the odds seem to go against them, especially when tiredness is a daily struggle. For example, it can be difficult to juggle the literature, others' and their own experiences with the supplements, and frequent fatigue and "brainfogginess" while at the same time trying to make sense of their genetic data with the thoroughness that seems to be necessary to make sense of this "complicated stuff." A member describes how she has reached a point of "stuckness," but has no option other than to continue. For many SNPNet members, this DIY-style route has been an economical choice and as she describes, with all the tests that are out there, she had to "choose wisely and economize."

In their efforts to learn, the members juggle a number of online database resources including public databases such as PubMed, OMIN, and dbSNP, and the online wiki SNPedia, but also spreadsheets and code developed by members of the community and others. Over time, there has been a shift in the use of these devices in line with growing lay expertise and interest in the practice. For people who have gone the "cheap" route, the first step is to work out what it means to be homozygous (both copies are mutated) or heterozygous (one copy is mutated) for the SNPs that are considered relevant to the treatment protocol. To begin, members would study SNPedia, published research papers, and Amy Yasko's sample report and her book to get some information on the thirty or so SNPs that are included in Yasko's genetic test, then compare these findings to their own "raw data" from 23andMe. Later, a member of SNPNet put these findings together onto a Google spreadsheet that was then used by the group. This spreadsheet was meant to help people who had done the 23andMe gene test to convert their SNP data into Yasko's format that interprets the alleles with the symbols plus or minus or both, rather than the chemical bases GACT. Through this move, a new, supposedly simpler standard was adopted that fits with Yasko's reports, although this conversion often proved to be rather problematic. A few months after, the task of translation had been delegated to a computer program developed by another of SNPNet's members who added color codes to the results: red for full defect, yellow for partial defect, and green for no defect (see figure 1.2). As a consequence, the work of analysis had become an automated task, blackboxed and further simplified in color codes. Prior to the use of the tools, members would discuss and sometimes struggle with these translations, but in the process build up an understanding of the complexity of the task and its exploratory nature, which later were formalized in spreadsheets and computer codes and in effect partly made invisible.

| Gene & Variation | rsID | Alleles | Result |
|---|---|---|---|
| COMT V158M | rs4680 | AG | +/- |
| COMT H62H | rs4633 | CT | +/- |
| COMT P199P | rs769224 | GG | -/- |
| VDR Bsm | rs1544410 | CT | +/- |
| VDR Taq | rs731236 | AG | +/- |
| MAO A R297R | rs6323 | TT | +/+ |
| ACAT1-02 | rs3741049 | AG | +/- |
| MTHFR C677T | rs1801133 | GG | -/- |
| MTHFR 03 P39P | rs2066470 | AG | +/- |
| MTHFR A1298C | rs1801131 | GT | +/- |
| MTR A2756G | rs1805087 | AA | -/- |
| MTRR A66G | rs1801394 | AG | +/- |
| MTRR H595Y | rs10380 | CC | -/- |
| MTRR K350A | rs162036 | AA | -/- |
| MTRR R415T | rs2287780 | CT | +/- |
| MTRR A664A | rs1802059 | GG | -/- |
| BHMT-02 | rs567754 | CT | +/- |
| BHMT-04 | rs617219 | AC | +/- |
| BHMT-08 | rs651852 | TT | +/+ |
| AHCY-01 | rs819147 | CT | +/- |
| AHCY-02 | rs819134 | AG | +/- |
| AHCY-19 | rs819171 | CT | +/- |
| CBS C699T | rs234706 | GG | -/- |
| CBS A360A | rs1801181 | AG | +/- |
| CBS N212N | rs2298758 | GG | -/- |
| SHMT1 C1420T | rs1979277 | GG | -/- |

**Figure 1.2**
Sample report. Source: SNPNet member's analysis tool, based on sample 23andMe data. Reprinted with permission.

Other applications have since appeared that also offer free detoxification reports in addition to extended versions provided for a fee ($20 to $37) and promoted to help individuals with their nutritional needs in an effort to "improve short and long term health, fitness and mental state" and "attain optimum health for yourself and your family" (e.g., LiveWello.com and Sterling's App from MTHFRsupport.com). Although the latest applications are not sold as treatment plans but as "nutritional guides" and "custom reports," the basic premise underlying these services is individual choice (Mol 2008). However, as we explore in the next sections, applications such as these can only provide individuals with directions that are managed through care-work and a process of "trial and error."

### Practicing Prediction and Prioritizing the Body

Just as the members have struggled with the translations, the group has also grappled with members' interpretations, and continues to do so.

Having worked out which SNPs could potentially be problematic and therefore need attention is no guarantee for a treatment plan. It may give them direction, but slowly, members are learning that prediction is not the basis for therapeutic action, but rather for negotiation and discussion that operates *alongside* the process of trial and error. Prediction is a process—not a starting point—that also involves learning a new "language." SNPNet members have for example suggested that there is "an order of healing," in other words, of which SNPs to target first. Members have also recommended that potential gut issues are addressed before taking any of the methylation supplements, especially if you have problems on the "cystathionine beta-synthase (CBS) pathway" (see figure 1.3 for a diagram of the methylation pathways).

Being homozygous on the CBS A360 mutation, for example, can cause problems as it is suggested that this mutation is an upregulation, which means that an increased CBS activity can lead to toxic sulphites being released in the body. This can cause chest tightness, nausea, and hives. Even with a heterozygous profile, Amy Yasko suggests that if one's "betaine homocysteine methyltransferase (BHMT) pathways" are defective, the CBS pathway is burdened to the extent that more sulfur and ammonia are created. Others disagree (e.g., Mark London [n.d.], who suffers

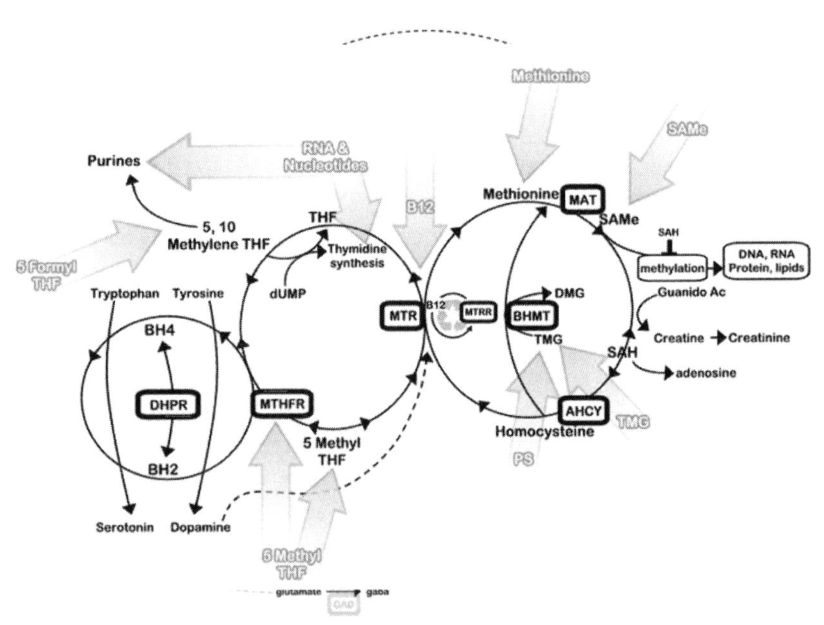


**Figure 1.3**
Methylation. Image courtesy of Dr Amy Yasko, Holistic Health International.

from fibromyalgia and has been researching and writing about the illness for many years). Taking Yasko's theory seriously, it is therefore important to "get the basics on board" before starting methylation. A member of SNPNet describes it as "cleaning up" before moving on to "fixing the genes" in order to avoid making "more garbage." But she also warns that although this might be what the literature suggests, it is crucial to take into account a person's illness history and level of sickness. The body must always be prioritized. Getting a basic feel for where you are when adding simple supplements and slowly learning their effects on the body is important, the member explains, because moving too quickly will most likely end "in crashing and lost time."

None of the SNPNet members can afford to leave aside the body, but rather, in order for them to learn, they need to tune into the body; they are, after all, as they put it, their own lab rats. Many have learned the hard way that hurrying up will lead to no good, but rather, treatment is precarious and disruptions cannot be avoided. Genetic testing, supplements, and predictions alone cannot be prescribed for the mending of a toxic body, which requires careful and persistent 'body work' and, not least, a lot of time. With diligence, the so-called path of healing might become more bearable. Living with a treatment protocol like Amy Yasko's, or versions of hers, is therefore not about compliance or adherence (e.g., Liza McCoy [2009] writes about adherence work for people living with HIV); rather, such a plan is continually negotiated and improvised, taking into consideration individual biographies, biomedical knowledge, advice from fellow SNPNet members, and not least the physical body. This biosensing practice shows that despite the availability of materials, the body fights back and cannot be ignored. Although the body is expected to resist the SNP data's partial conclusions and the treatment protocol's directions, it is nevertheless a necessary process of trial and error that cannot be resolved with more data and more (incomplete) biomedical knowledge. Biosensing is an improvised and embodied practice (e.g., see Mol and Law [2004] on hypoglycemia as an embodied action).

This genetic data practice in some ways exemplifies what Dana Greenfield (chapter 7, this volume) calls the *n of 1*—an experimental system, she argues, where the focus is on knowledge gained at the scale of the individual. There is no requirement for large numbers, statistical validity, or expert credentials, but instead, it is a space "where new possibilities for the meaning and experience of health and illness ramify in surprising ways." *N of 1* is a starting place, she writes, for "thinking outside given frameworks of what is normal and abnormal." Practicing prediction might well be part of such experimental system.

**What's in a Promise?**

The potential of direct-to-consumer genetic testing creates a sense of hope, despite the work required. It gives SNPNet members something to look forward to and it creates excitement. Hope is part of what makes them want to learn and dig into the world of methylation, biochemistry, and supplements, despite the fact that it can take months to learn and requires a good amount of effort. But this in part also contributes to the hope, at least for some of the members, in that there now is a plan, not necessarily a treatment plan, but a plan for moving forward. They show consideration and care for each other and for the complex and often difficult tasks at hand. This motivates hope. Some, for example, struggle to concentrate on the reading and video material, let alone knowing what an SNP is. Others then offer to help, but also point out that over time it will become "more understandable." This temporal horizon or duration plays a key part in this bio-sensing practice in that it helps to maintain a sense of hope. But at the same time, practicing hope in this way can also be understood as a form of seduction in that it persuades people to keep searching for the answers to their health concerns. This presupposes that there *is* an answer to be found and as long as we keep looking, as long as we keep up the "good work," we *will* find it. It can easily become a search for that piece of the puzzle that will explain everything. Yasko (2004) herself claims to have found that piece, not only for children with autism, but also, she asserts, her program could "prove effective" for conditions such as Alzheimer's disease, chronic fatigue syndrome, fibromyalgia, and ADHD. Promises like those made by Amy Yasko of "optimized health" and "proven results" can be hard to ignore, even more so for those who desperately seek help.

On SNPNet, however, the only promise made is that time, effort, and resources are required to learn how to make sense of the genetic data, methylation and detoxification reports, and the (scientific) literature, and those understandings can easily be disrupted by new findings and experiences. Predictions, supplement recommendations, and the illusion of control are (eventually) all put into practice and worked on in their incompleteness. What to do next is not as straightforward as described in any treatment protocol, but fraught with ambivalence that can only be resolved, momentarily, through trial and error. Deeply involved in this data practice, members learn that the treatment plan on paper will never work in practice, but it can only provide direction and somewhere to start. From there, the individual works with the ambivalence and the incompleteness of biomedical knowledge to figure out what works best for her at a given time. These are incorporated into and become an essential part of the attempts to get better through trial and error. Ambivalence and the incompleteness of biomedical knowledge are therefore not only what brings this group of people together, but also what takes them forward. Uncertainty has a kind of material force (see Franklin and Roberts [2006] on how uncertainty can create reassurance and trust and be made to "account" for technologies; Singleton and Michael [1993] on how ambiguity and instability can contribute to a technology's continuation). Although, in this practice, learning about the body necessarily encounters instability, the ambivalence and incompleteness are precisely made manageable because this is done with care. Making sense of the plurality of materials matters through its sociality. Having others to discuss and negotiate, disagree and agree with—or simply to share one's genetic testing results and medical literature with—makes the uncertainties more bearable. This is care. It is a way "to handle unfolding uncertainties that are also in tension in a way that holds them together imperfectly" (Law et al. 2014, 183). Others have argued for the management of biomedical uncertainty through the creation of technoscientific identities (Sulik 2009) or through acts of love and affection (Silverman 2012).

## Concluding Remarks

We have suggested that DNA microarray-based biosensing sharply poses the question of whether biosensors biomedicalize. Microarray genotyping is characterized by the leveraging and assembling of a plurality of forms, standards, knowledge, technologies, and practices that support the care of data. It depends on the computer and statistical sciences to recognize patterns of variations and to highlight possible associations. As commodities, microarrays build on molecular biology and genomics, robotics and automation. They overflow the clinical institutions of biomedicine, but flow into the domain of the marketization of science and the commodification of health. These developments make up a rich technoscientific practice that appears to fit the biomedicalization thesis (Clarke et al. 2003). The DNA biosensor is technoscientifically engineered; it is part of new organizational and informational infrastructures; it extends healthcare knowledge production, distribution, and information management sites to include the market, the Internet, and the home; it is also a cultural device in that social forms and spaces are coproduced with science and technology; and it is a device used to offer people a service good that is imagined to help them minimize, manage, and treat disease and health risks.

Does DNA-based biosensing biomedicalize? "Yes" is the short answer. However, although the biomedicalization thesis provides an expansive account of contemporary biomedicine, the DNA-based biosensing practice that is explored in this chapter sits slightly uncomfortably within the biomedicalization thesis. None of its tools can account for the intrinsic instability that pervades the practice, ranging from DNA's sensitivity to biological processes around it to the uncertainty that pervades the practices of sensemaking. DNA-based biosensors come with their own set of instabilities that biomedicalization only partly explains.

Learning which questions to ask and which materials to access and how to use them can be hard work. A slow learning process that takes time, effort, and resources. It is an improvised practice that leads to partial answers that will hold for a while until disrupted by new findings and experiences, more (incomplete) biomedical knowledge, and new tools and computer programs. Also, and important, the body is not simply a project, but is also prioritized all the way through in a process of "trial and error" that best describes this DNA-based biosensing practice. The instabilities encountered when learning about the body and the treatment protocol's uncertainties are managed precisely because this is done with care—not simply self-care, but also care for each other. Learning to make sense, practicing prediction, and prioritizing the body are not simply individual undertakings, but also shared, collective acts of care that makes the uncertainties more bearable. These social spaces of care therefore come to interfere with the biomedicalization processes that more broadly focus on individual moral responsibilities fulfilled through access to knowledge, self-surveillance, and consumption of biomedical goods and services.

Yet, despite the acts of (good) care, what happens to people in these instances of biosensing? Is this group of people relieved from or subjected to (more) suffering? Empowered or seduced? If biosensing comes with the potential to transform bodies, in situations of care where the desperate and the rational go hand in hand, the burden of not taking action can quickly instigate a downward spiral of more suffering. Also, if DNA-based biosensing exemplifies the broader scope of medical practice to include the commodification of health and the promotion of self-care, then this could further sustain and occlude the lack of care provided by the medical community. The availability of biomedical goods and services and biomedical knowledge does not automatically improve care. As Mol (2008, 2) writes in her book *The Logic of Care*, "[p]atient choice ... does not (finally) make space for us, its patient," and therefore rather than "dreaming of choice, it is better to improve care on its own terms." These questions are not meant as a terminal critique of biosensors, but rather are intended to disturb some of their potential consequences and open up discussion of their socialities.

## Acknowledgments

The SNPNet study forms part of Kragh-Furbo's doctoral dissertation on genetic data practices in consumer genomics and is nested within the wider project Living Data: Making Sense of Health Biosensors.

## Notes

1. BRCA1/2 tests are full-sequence tests done by either multiplexed quantitative PCR (polymerase chain reaction) or microarray-CGH (comparative genomics hybridization) analysis (Myriad Genetic Laboratories 2012).

2. The DNA sequences on the microarrays can be detected via laser-excited fluorescent stains. High-resolution images of visible differences are recorded using confocal microscopy technology (Inoué 2006).

3. Transducers are devices to convert a component of the sample (analyte) into a measurable physical signal.

4. See UCSC Genome Bioinformatics website https://genome.ucsc.edu/.

## References

ACMG. 2008. "Policy Statement on Direct-to-Consumer Genetic Testing." https://www.acmg.net/. Accessed March 6, 2014.

Arribas-Ayllon, Michael, Katie Featherstone, and Paul Atkinson. 2011. "The Practical Ethics of Genetic Responsibility: Non-Disclosure and the Autonomy of Affect." *Social Theory & Health* 9 (1): 3–23.

Banica, Florinel-Gabriel. 2012. *Chemical Sensors and Biosensors: Fundamentals and Applications*. West Sussex, UK: John Wiley & Sons, Ltd..

Burton, P. R., D. G. Clayton, L. R. Cardon, N. Craddock, P. Deloukas, A. Duncanson, A. Kwiatkowski, 2007. "Genome-wide Association Study of 14,000 Cases of Seven Common Diseases and 3,000 Shared Controls." *Nature* 447 (June): 661–678. doi:10.1038/nature05911.

Chua, A., C. Y. Yean, M. Ravichandran, B. Lim, and P. Lalitha. 2011. "A Rapid DNA Biosensor for the Molecular Diagnosis of Infectious Disease." *Biosensors & Bioelectronics* 26 (9): 3825–3831.

Clarke, A. E., J. K. Shim, L. Mamo, J. R. Fosket, and J. R. Fishman. 2003. "Biomedicalization: Technoscientific Transformations of Health, Illness, and U.S. Biomedicine." *American Sociological Review* 68 (2): 161–194. doi:10.2307/1519765.

Curnutte, Margaret, and Giuseppe Testa. 2012. "Consuming Genomes: Scientific and Social Innovation in Direct-to-Consumer Genetic Testing." *New Genetics & Society* 31 (2): 159–181.

Delfanti, Alessandra. 2012. Tweaking Genes in Your Garage: Biohacking between Activism and Entrepreneurship. In *Activist Media and Biopolitics: Critical Media Interventions in the Age of Biopower*, ed. Wolfgang Sützl and Theo Hug, 163–178. Innsbruck, Austria: Innsbruck University Press.

EASAC. 2012. "Direct-to-Consumer Genetic Testing for Health-related Purposes in the European Union: The view from EASAC and FEAM." http://www.easac.eu/home/reports-and-statements/detail-view/article/direct-to-co.html. Accessed March 6, 2014.

Encode Consortium. 2012. "An Integrated Encyclopedia of DNA Elements in the Human Genome." *Nature* 489 (September): 57–74. doi:10.1038/nature11247.

Foster, Morris, John Mulvihill, and Richard R. Sharp. 2009. "Evaluating the Utility of Personal Genomic Information." *Genetics in Medicine* 11 (8): 570–574.

Franklin, Sarah, and Celia Roberts. 2006. *Born and Made: An Ethnography of Preimplantation Genetic Diagnosis*. Oxfordshire: Princeton University Press.

Groenen, P. J. F., A. Hofman, P. Koellinger, M. van der Loos, F. Rivadeneira, F. van Rooij, R. Thurik, and A. Uitterlinden. 2008. "Genome-Wide Association for Loci Influencing Entrepreneurial Behavior: The Rotterdam Study." *Behavior Genetics* 38 (6): 628–629.

Groves, Chris, and Richard Tutton. 2013. "Walking the Tightrope: Expectations and Standards in Personal Genomics." *Biosocieties* 8 (2): 181–204.

Hauskeller, Christine. 2011. "Direct to Consumer Genetic Testing: Regulations Cannot Guarantee Responsible Use; An International Industry Certificate Is Needed." *British Medical Journal (Clinical Research Ed.)* 342 (April): d2317. doi:10.1136/bmj.d2317.

Howard, Heidi Carmen, and Pascal Borry. 2012. "To Ban or Not to Ban?" *EMBO Reports* 13 (9): 791–794.

Inoué, Shinya. 2006. Foundations of Confocal Scanned Imaging in Light Microscopy. In *Handbook of Biological Confocal Microscopy*, ed. James B. Pawley, 1–19. New York: Springer.

The International HapMap Consortium. 2005. "A Haplotype Map of the Human Genome." *Nature* 437 (October): 1299–1320. doi:10.1038/nature04226.

Jolie, A. 2013. "My Medical Choice." *New York Times*, May 14. http://www.nytimes.com/2013/05/14/opinion/my-medical-choice.html. Accessed March 11, 2014.

Keller, E. F. 2000. *The Century of the Gene*. Cambridge, MA: Harvard University Press.

Kerr, Anne. 2004. *Genetics and Society: A Sociology of Disease*. London: Routledge.

Langreth, Robert, and John Lauerman. 2012. "Autism Cures Promised by DNA Testers Belied by Regulators." Bloomberg News, December 21. http://www.bloomberg.com/news/2012-12-21/autism-cures-promised-by-dna-testers-belied-by-regulators.html. Accessed April 7, 2014.

Lave, Jean, and Etienne Wenger. 1991. *Situated Learning: Legitimate Peripheral Participation*. Cambridge: Cambridge University Press.

Law, John, Geir Afdal, Kristin Asdal, Ingunn Moser, and Vicky Singleton. 2014. "Modes of Syncretism: Notes on Noncoherence." *Common Knowledge* 20 (1): 172–192.

Levina, Marina. 2010. "Googling Your Genes: Personal Genomics and the Discourse of Citizen Bioscience in the Network Age." *Journal of Science Communication* 9 (1): 1–8.

London, Mark R. n.d. "CBS Upregulation, Myth or Reality." http://web.mit.edu/london/www/cbs.html. Accessed March 5, 2014.

O'Riordan, Kate. 2010. *The Genome Incorporated: Constructing Biodigital Identity*. Farnham, UK: Ashgate Publishing Limited.

McCoy, Liza. 2009. "Time, Self and Medication Day: A Closer Look at the Everyday Work of 'Adherence.'" *Sociology of Health & Illness* 31 (1): 128–146.

McGuire, Amy, and Wylie Burke. 2008. "An Unwelcome Side Effect of Direct-to-Consumer Personal Genome Testing." *Journal of the American Medical Association* 300 (22): 2669–2671.

Mol, Annemarie. 2008. *The Logic of Care: Health and the Problems of Patient Choice*. Oxon: Routledge.

Mol, Annemarie, and John Law. 2004. "Embodied Action, Enacted Bodies: An Example of Hypoglycaemia." *Body & Society* 10 (2–3): 43–62.

Myriad Genetic Laboratories. 2012. BRAC*Analysis* Technical Specifications. https://www.myriad.com/lib/technical-specifications/BRACAnalysis-Technical-Specifications.pdf. Accessed July 31, 2015.

Schena, M., D. Shalon, R. W. Davis, and P. O. Brown. 1995. "Quantitative Monitoring of Gene Expression Patterns with a Complementary DNA Microarray." *Science* 270 (5235): 467–470. doi:10.1126/science.270.5235.467.

Shi, L., G. Campbell, W. D. Jones, F. Campagne, Z. Wen, S. J. Walker, Z. Su, 2010. "The MicroArray Quality Control (MAQC)-II Study of Common Practices for the Development and Validation of Microarray-Based Predictive Models." *Nature Biotechnology* 28 (8): 827–838. doi:10.1038/nbt.1665.

Silverman, Chloe. 2012. *Understanding Autism: Parents, Doctors, and the History of a Disorder*. Princeton, NJ: Princeton University Press.

Singleton, Vicky, and Mike Michael. 1993. "Actor-Networks and Ambivalence: General Practitioners in the UK Cervical Screening Programme." *Social Studies of Science* 23 (2): 227–264.

Siva, Nayanah. 2008. "1000 Genomes Project." *Nature Biotechnology* 26 (3): 256. doi:10.1038/nbt0308-256b.

Spencer, David H., and Christina Lockwood. 2011. "Direct-to-Consumer Genetic Testing: Reliable or Risky?" *Clinical Chemistry* 57 (12): 1641–1644.

Stevens, H. 2013. *Life Out of Sequence: A Data-Driven History of Bioinformatics*. Chicago, London: University Of Chicago Press.

Sulik, Gayle A. 2009. "Managing Biomedical Uncertainty: The Technoscientific Illness Identity." *Sociology of Health & Illness* 30 (7): 1059–1076.

Szymczak, S., J. M. Biernacka, H. J. Cordell, O. González-Recio, I. R. König, H. Zhang, and Y. V. Sun. 2009. "Machine Learning in Genome-wide Association Studies." *Genetic Epidemiology* 33 (suppl 1): S51–S57.

Thiruppathiraja, C., S. Kamatchiammal, P. Adaikkappan, D. J. Santhosh, and M. Alagar. 2011. "Specific Detection of Mycobacterium Sp. Genomic DNA Using Dual Labeled Gold Nanoparticle Based Electrochemical Biosensor." *Analytical Biochemistry* 417 (1): 73–79.

23andMe. 2013. "23andMe's New Custom Chip." November 18. http://blog.23andme.com/news/23andmes-new-custom-chip/. Accessed September 2, 2014.

Yang, J., B. Benyamin, B. P. McEvoy, S. Gordon, A. K. Henders, D. R. Nyholt, P. A. Madden, 2010. "Common SNPs Explain a Large Proportion of the Heritability for Human Height." *Nature Genetics* 42 (7): 565–569. doi:10.1038/ng.608.

Yasko, Amy. 2004. *Autism: Pathways to Recovery*. Bethel, ME: Neurological Research Institute.

# 2

# Data in the Age of Digital Reproduction: Reading the Quantified Self through Walter Benjamin

Jamie Sherman

## Prologue: Walter Benjamin Takes the Measure of Art

Walter Benjamin, writing in Europe a few short years before World War II, argued that improvements in the technical reproduction of images and the rise of film were having a profound impact on society. For Benjamin, the nature of the shift from print to lithograph to photograph to film was an acceleration of speed and intensity. Works of art, Benjamin noted, had always been reproducible, but at much slower speeds, in both the production of the copy through manual means, and in its distribution.

In his essay "The Work of Art in the Age of Mechanical Reproduction," Benjamin's argument is not that photographs and film cannot be art, a debate he calls "futile," and "confused" (1968, 226). Rather, he insists that the mechanisms of mass reproduction change something fundamental about art itself. First, they detach the artwork from the physical object, situated in space and time. Whereas in more manual art forms, the work of art and its physical articulation in an object are one and the same, in film and photography, where copies abound, the artwork is distinct from any given copy of it (220). Second, this dislocation undermines the aura of specificity that had historically been vested in art, in favor of a "sense of the universal equality of things" (223). No copy is more or less original than another; rather, all copies are equal, and therefore largely interchangeable. Third, for Benjamin, the twentieth-century unhinging of art from the constraints of singularity, through reproduction, and presence, through distribution, uproots art from its original place in cult and ritual. Fourth, Benjamin argues that this new era of cult-free art makes art available to—and vulnerable to—other social categories, particularly the politics of fascism and communism as they played out in Europe in the lead up to World War II (224). Later scholars, notably Baudrillard, link images detached from any "original" to consumer capitalism in ways that Benjamin does not, but that resonate well with Benjamin's basic framework (Baudrillard 1994).

Reading Benjamin's essay nearly a century after it was written, parallels between images in the twentieth century and data in the twenty-first are striking. We, too, find ourselves at a moment of acceleration that feels emergent and profound, promising and ominous, with repercussions on our social and cultural systems we have yet to understand. Humans have been counting and measuring and tracking things for millennia, and yet the speed, depth, and breadth of this enumeration have undergone, and are undergoing, a process of rapid transformation. It seems at the very least likely, if not entirely certain, that the acceleration of data is changing something about how life is measured, counted, and made accountable, and what kinds of things matter in a more measured world.

This chapter draws on Benjamin's discussion of the mechanisms of image capture and distribution as a lens through which to view the current moment. While there is a larger picture and question out there in relation to "big data" this essay focuses on the specific question of data and the self, drawing on ethnographic fieldwork within the Quantified Self community, primarily on the West Coast of the United States.

The Quantified Self community, founded by Gary Wolf and Kevin Kelly in 2007, is described on their website as "an international collaboration of users and makers of self-tracking tools" dedicated to helping "people get meaning out of their personal data." Primarily volunteer run, local leaders in about a hundred cities across thirty countries organize "meetups" where participants are invited to present stories about their experiences with personal data tracking in a format they call "show and tell."

Within the Quantified Self (or QS) community, and in this chapter, data are understood in very broad terms. Generally speaking, personal data are things measured or recorded (tracked) or both in some way shape or form; most often, though not always, this form is digital. Many folks within QS use spreadsheets. Many of them also use devices and software applications that either take measurements and record information independently (e.g., a pedometer), or prompt the person to enter information at various times of day (e.g., many "mood" trackers). Quite a few use both, or all three.

The point of the exercise, viewing data in the Quantified Self through the lens of Benjamin, is less about presenting a coherent argument about the sameness of data and film, our moment in history and Benjamin's, than it is about opening up a range of questions and perhaps insights regarding what that comparison reveals. In particular, it draws our attention to the representational aspect of data, the role and function of abstraction in QS, and the mechanisms through which data as representation and abstraction restructure lived experience. Finally, it raises questions about the ways that the acceleration, or expansion of data into the realm of the self might be understood as a domain shift analogous to the movement of art into politics and economics.

## Four Months, Seventy-eight Years: Michael Cohn's Quantified Self and "That Guy"

On a rainy night in late March of 2014, four months before rereading Benjamin's essay, and some seventy-eight years after it was written, I attended an event organized by the Bay Area Quantified Self meetup group. We gathered in a large gallery at the San Francisco Exploratorium, overlooking the bay, on folding chairs arranged in an arc facing a podium and a screen. There were four presentations. In the first of these, Michael Cohn,[1] a graduate student in psychology, talked about his use of spreadsheets and a system of "irrational commitment" that helped him regulate his behavior (see Cohn 2014). Cohn described his problem in terms of "this guy," shown in the slides as a shadowy, red-tinted image of Michael himself. "This guy," he told us, doesn't care about his other commitments or his desire to live a healthier life. "He" wants instant gratification and cares little for Michael's concerns about mental and physical health, job performance, and professional achievement. "He" stays up late playing video games though he know Michael needs to work, eats junk food though Michael is trying to eat healthier, and generally undermines Michael's efforts to manage his life in keeping with his goals for himself. Michael told us that by creating specific goals (I will work on *x* project for at least *y* amount of time), and then tracking his actual behavior relevant to those goals in spreadsheets he creates each week, he was better able to limit the effects of "that guy." It works, he said, because the concrete nature of those commitments was something "that guy" could understand and left no "wiggle room."

Thinking about Benjamin, it suddenly comes to seem significant, or at least poignant, that Michael uses a photograph to represent the undesirable aspects of himself in lieu of any other possible way he might have chosen. "That guy" is not Michael, exactly, but rather some aspect or part of himself at odds with the rest. Michael's data consisted of multiple spreadsheets tracking commitments set, and values placed on fulfilling those commitments in terms of done/not done and in increments of time (minutes spent being "productive" or at the gym, for example). Over time, Michael told us, he added more and more categories to his weekly array of commitments that shift and change in relation to his activities and preoccupations at any given time. In this way, Michael's story constructed an unfolding of himself in both data and image. In image, "that guy" contrasted with the articulate, well-groomed graduate student standing at the front of the room. In data, Michael's spreadsheets traced an ongoing process of thresholds, standards, and measurements that bound the two together, Michael the graduate student setting the parameters and recording that guy's compliance. The data became a drama depicting an inner battle between his better self and the selfish other guy, where victories, defeats, and consequences played out in numbers, lists, and time kept.

At the moment of this writing, when selfies are circulated through an ever-expanding range of mobile devices and platforms, images and data are hopelessly tangled; images as a kind of data are largely interchangeable with other kinds of data distributed through open and closed networks, stored in bits and bytes. Against the backdrop of that entanglement, the blending of data and image in Michael's presentation surfaces parallel questions of how selfies and self-tracking relate to the selves they represent.

## Proximity and Distance: Auras and Operations

For Benjamin, the relationship between image and imaged is central to understanding where photography moves radically away from prior forms of visual representation. Fundamentally, filmic images and their widespread distribution reconfigure relationships of proximity and distance that bind a thing (or person) to the quality that make it uniquely itself, what Benjamin calls the "aura."

Aura, for Benjamin is a function of singularity and presence. It is the quality of an object, a place, or a person that one can only experience in the presence of the original. He uses the example of seeing a mountain and being struck by the beauty and majesty of the view. The power of the landscape (actual, not painted) is in its presence, which one can perceive only from sufficient distance to take the whole thing in (singularity), and only in person—you have to be there (presence). Thus aura, in Benjamin, entails both the relative distance of a vantage point, and the relative proximity in having to be present in some contiguous space and time.

"Manually produced" works of art, such as paintings, have such an aura of singularity for Benjamin. There is only one authentic Mona Lisa, for example, and she can only be truly experienced by being present at the Louvre, in the gallery where she hangs on the wall. Photographic images, however, lack an aura of their own; they appear as transparent renditions of their objects, while failing to capture the aura of those things. Images of the Mona Lisa encountered elsewhere in photographs or film are but pale copies. Further, for Benjamin, the ubiquity of copies, poster versions of the Mona Lisa hanging in living rooms and doctor offices across the globe, leach from the Mona Lisa her uniqueness and historical specificity—her aura—in ways that make the Mona Lisa hanging at the Louvre seem but little more than a copy of herself.

Citing the many ways that film captures details not available to the naked eye, or too quick for human perception, Benjamin argues that the cameraman penetrates the photographic subject in ways he likens to a surgeon cutting into the body of a patient with a focus on the operation rather than the patient as a person (1968, 233). The resultant product, the film or photograph, consists of "multiple fragments which are assembled under a new law" of photographic production and reproduction. By contrast, the "painter maintains in his work a natural distance from reality," and the representation produced by a painter, is "a total one" (Benjamin 1968, 233–234). In this sense, then, photographic images are, for Benjamin, too close to their subject.

At the same time that images are, for Benjamin, too close to the person or thing captured to render a holistic representation, the mechanisms of reproduction and distribution also render the subject too far. If the aura of a person, an artwork, a particular view can only be encountered through locatedness in a single space-time, multiplicity (a thing that exists in multiple, distributed copies) disrupts this relationship. Photographs are too close, in the sense that they are the result of a surgeon-like focus on detail, and too far in the sense that one encounters their subjects from a distance, disjunctive in space and time.

While one might argue with Benjamin over the relationship between painters, photographers, and their respective subjects, his analogy is provocative in relation to data collection. Data collection, however idiosyncratic, tends to approach the thing measured or recorded (whether happiness, productivity, intimacy, or fluid levels) through attention to separable details. Minutes stand in for activity, steps stand in for fitness, food is captured through particular ratios of fat, sugars, and fiber.

## Fragmentation and Wholes: Differentiation and Commensurability

Unlike people and paintings, actions and experiences frequently lack clear boundaries that distinguish them as a whole (or wholes). Experiences bleed into one another in ways that are decidedly fuzzy. Thus while measuring material things in the world such as bottles of wine, or counting people at the level of population is fairly straightforward, measuring experiences like mood, productivity, or even fitness demands an imposition of boundaries and a definition of parameters. Like Benjamin's photographs, these parameters (minutes, scales, laps) capture aspects of the thing measured; unlike photographs, the measurement also redefines the object of measurement as a thing in itself, as well as selecting it as proxy for the larger abstraction it is understood to capture (steps as a measure of fitness, for example). While photographs, for Benjamin, fail to approach their subjects as a whole, focusing instead on specific details, or facets, that then come to appear as if whole, data collection has the capacity to create the boundaries that define the whole it represents through the proxy of aspects measured.

Michael's understanding of what did and did not constitute periods of productive writing differentiated those moments from the broader flow of moment to moment in his life, and reframed them as something—as productive writing—in contrast to other kinds of things Michael might have been engaged in. In fact, Michael was not very specific about how such moments were defined: what was "productive writing" in contrast to other kinds of possible activities? Yet, even in the absence of a precise definition (perhaps he knew it when he felt it), recording those minutes bound them together and differentiated them from the rest. Whereas the "original" that film captures—whether it is a person, a mountain, or a work of art has, for Benjamin, a prior existence as a singular whole, when self-tracking turns its attention to experience, or behavior, the tracking itself has the capacity to define and produce the thing measured.

Yet Benjamin's discussion of auras as related to their unreproducibility is akin to, if not the same as, the unreproducibility of experience. One day's writing can be experientially quite different from the next, each with its own sequence and array of thoughts, feelings, itches, hunches, distractions, epiphanies, and ellipses. The designation of a time as "productive writing" serves to capture an aspect of it (that it was in some sense "productive") while eliding those nuances that made it uniquely those moments and not any other. In other words, measuring and tracking in the ways that constitute data in the QS community do not capture the incommensurability of experience. In fact, it is largely by bracketing out that incommensurability (the aura of a moment, we might say, bending Benjamin to our own purposes) that data works. By abstracting from the day particular moments, and designating them "productive," Michael is able to compare experiences that are otherwise not really comparable.

Benjamin's complaint, then, that the lack of aura in photographs undermines specificity in favor of a "sense of the universal equality of things" (Benjamin 1968, 223) is precisely what makes data useful. Bounding certain experiences off from the flow of one moment to the next, and capturing them in ways that make them commensurate is how datasets "work."

Seen this way, Michael's efforts to manage his productivity and his behavior over time using the photographic image of "this guy" make constructive use of the parallels between photographs and data as abstractions that both capture and create distance. The image of "this guy" renders visible a mental image, perhaps, by means of which Michael exorcises those qualities and behaviors that "this guy" represents in ways that sever "this guy" from Michael; the murky reddish "selfie" captures and contains those aspects of Michael's self-image that he hopes to abstract through the practices of data tracking. Thus the image of "this guy," too close in Benjamin's terms, captures details of Michael that do not, ultimately, add up to Michael as a whole, but through its fragmentation lend Michael a vantage point from which to view these aspects of himself. Michael's self-tracking project sutures together Michael's commitments and Michael's fulfillment or failure through fragments of Michael measured. By measuring "this guy's" time and check boxes, Michael abstracts action from experience in time spent, workouts accomplished, or pages written that likewise create a sort of composite representation of a larger whole that is only ever partly captured (Benjamin's surgical penetration), but that gives Michael a vantage point from which to view and—importantly for Michael—to manage his behavior.

## Mechanisms and Facticity

Benjamin argues that some of the power of film and photography lies in the way they seem like a window onto the reality they capture. Benjamin suggests that this transparency is produced through the elision within the image of the means of its production. He points to the fact that film and photography are highly technical and equipment intensive with lights, meters, tripods, and other devices that do not appear in the image. Whereas painting clearly reveals itself as representational through brushstrokes and other indicators of the medium and the labor through which it was produced, film and photography hide that mechanism and thus appear as if transparent. This argument is, once again, provocative in relation to data, evoking the ways that categories of data (such as "steps" in current activity trackers) appear not only as a transparent capture of a particular fact of having taken (or not taken) a specific number of steps that day, but also—as importantly—as a proxy for having achieved (or failed to achieve) a level of "activity." The mechanisms for the collection of those data, the particular sensor and the algorithms through which it translates its sensing into a measurement, disappear behind the number in ways that give the number a sense of facticity—a window onto reality.

Within QS, where participants are both measurer and measured, this tension plays out in interesting ways. At the level of data collection and data analysis, the specificity of the mechanism of data collection is significant, particularly to the person attempting to integrate various data "streams" to their own ends. Several of the breakout sessions at the 2012 Bay Area QS Conference and even more of those at the 2013 QS Conference in Amsterdam, discussed challenges associated with combining data streams from different devices, or even different spreadsheets, and in one presentation a man compared an array of activity trackers on the market at the time, while attendees debated the relative accuracy and the differences in how data were collected and interpreted by the devices. However, it is also true that debates regarding the accuracy of particular devices are like debates about camera lenses: photographers may passionately debate the appropriate lens for particular subjects under specific lighting conditions, but arguments about lenses do not question the basic relationship between the camera and the person or thing photographed. Similarly, debates about accuracy, while they may undermine particular devices, or even some datasets, do not question the basic relationship between measurement and measured as a capturing of some kind of facticity. Further, because datasets are in large part comparative projects (last month vs. this month, yesterday in relation to today), even arbitrary, made up numbers, so long as they are consistent, take on a particular sense of facticity. Using Nike's FuelBand, it doesn't matter that the fuel points do not equate to anything in particular, but the fact that I "earned" eight points today and only six points yesterday is understood and experienced as capturing some kind of fact regarding the relative activity over the course of two days.

The facility with which QS participants can discuss, often in great detail, the mechanisms and parameters of their tracking, and at the same time slip seamlessly into analyses that take the facticity of these measurements for granted is not a failure of comprehension or intelligence, but rather a testament to the powerful ways that the processes of measuring and tracking work to structure and construct facts from the flow of experience.

## Idiosyncratic Data, Quirky Commensurability

While many Quantified Self projects draw on measurements and parameters that are fairly common (e.g., weight, activity, or nutrition tracking) many other QS projects and experiments are remarkably idiosyncratic. The challenge of defining parameters to measure and then further developing a method for measuring them is far from obvious or standard in many cases. In one memorable encounter at the 2013 QS conference in Amsterdam, for example, a participant named Fabio told me that he had been feeling like the time and effort he was putting into relationships with various people in his life was not consistent with the relative importance of those relationships to him (see dos Santos 2015). Unimportant people were taking up too much time, and close relationships were getting short shrift. He began tracking all his interactions with people, new and old, in a small notebook. He showed me his entry for me. In a process that had clearly evolved over time, his notation included my name, a number designating how many minutes we spoke, and a symbol indicating that I had initiated the conversation, which I had done with a casual remark about the conference as we stood next to each other, two strangers, outside the main auditorium.[2] In addition to recording interactions, Fabio began keeping a list of the people in his life with a scale of their importance to him, using a combined score across three "indexes" including "Fi" or "Friendship index," "Ai" or "Attraction index," and "Bi" or "Business index" that together comprised the cleverly named "FABi" or Fabio index of that person in his life. Tracking these data, he told me, allowed him to more deliberately limit his engagements with people to whom his relationship was less critical, and also led to shifts in the ways he managed close relationships. In particular, he realized that by proactively reaching out to his mother, with whom he lived, he was better able to satisfy her desire for contact with him, while also limiting the number of interruptions from her that he had found annoying. In this way he felt that the tracking had helped him better his relationship to his mother.

Fabio's project, like Michael's, is in many ways quirky and distinctive and impressively creative. It is also, from a distance, rather uncomfortable for its ranking of people in ways that seem to reduce human relationships to a number, emptied of the particularities that make a person and a relationship unique. At the same time, that abstraction was what enabled Fabio to reprioritize his time in ways that were more in keeping with the relationships that meant something to him. For both Fabio's and Michael's purposes, the quirks of their evaluative systems, once in place, faded to the background and what mattered for their efficacy was the mechanism of measurement and abstraction, and the ways this process enabled commensurability between elements that otherwise were not comparable.

As discussed earlier in relation to facts, this play between comparable and not comparable plays out at the level of devices as well (see also Estrin and Hanika, chapter 9; Böhlen, chapter 10, and Taylor, chapter 11, this volume). Different devices use different sensors and different algorithms to translate motions sensed into a unit often glossed as "steps." The "steps" of one device are often not, strictly speaking and at the level of data, commensurate with those of another. Indeed, in a conversation last year with an entrepreneur who was working on a tracking application intended to work across Android-powered phones, I was told that the same application on the same operating system but different hardware (in this case different phone models) were often neither commensurate nor compatible. While several Quantified Self projects have undertaken comparisons between devices, it is notable that, generally speaking, steps from one device are seen as more or less the same as those from another. In other words, despite the "quirkiness" that can make data technically incommensurate across projects and devices, data tend to enact commensurability and comparability in the lives of people who use it.

Not only do steps abstract activity from the particular walk, run, stroll, or hike that they capture, they become commensurate across people, places, and time. My 10,000 steps today are not only comparable to my 10,000 steps yesterday, but also to my brother's steps, though he lives in another city and has a longer physical stride. Likewise, and despite the fact that my own criteria for what is and is not a "productive writing" moment may differ from Michael's, those of us in the audience were so easily able to think across our own experiences that a laugh of recognition rippled across the audience at his introduction. Our own efforts to each contain our own impulsive "this guy" were easily imagined in relation to his. Likewise, once Fabio began to describe how his ranking system helped him better balance his time as a reflection of his connection, it was easy to see how my own intimacies might benefit from a recalibration.

In part, perhaps, this kind of recognition was a result of shared cultural constructs that have come to emphasize "productivity" as something for individuals as well as industries to strive for, and intimacies as something to be managed. But I am suggesting here that the mechanisms of data as a process of abstraction enable commensurability and comparability across individual lives in ways that operate alongside and even independently of the particular criteria by which those things are measured. More, I am suggesting that the mechanisms of abstraction applied to experience this way begin to restructure not only that flow, but also the stories we tell ourselves about ourselves (see Geertz 1975, 448).

## Data, Presence, and Becoming

Toward the end of his presentation, Michael made a curious quasi-confession. Quantification, he told us, isn't really about the data for him. He has lots of data but, in fact, he hasn't "really figured out what to do with it." Instead, he said, quantification for him is about what it does for him "in the moment." While many Quantified Self participants do in fact perform data analysis, Michael's experience, the efficacy he finds in the act of self-tracking and even the lack of certainty about "what to do with it," is not uncommon. In addition, the siloing of data within apps and device platforms means that even technically savvy self-trackers frequently have limited access to data that can at times be distributed across several different locations. Thus, for many, the practice of tracking and collecting data is as far as things go. Yet the mental model of data as something you "do something with" where that "something" involves some kind of analytics is pervasive. Thus in the Quantified Self community there is often something of a gap between how people talk about data in terms of the things that they wish for or imagine they could do or will be able to do one day (if only, like Michael, they knew what to do with it or, alternately, could get it all together in the same place), and how data are used and experienced by many in the present—as what it does for them "in the moment."

The tone of Michael's statement, as well as its substance, speaks to collective assumptions regarding if not what data are, then what they are for. Data are implicitly posited as a kind of "raw" material that leads to an end product, with the dual implication of being intended for processing, and in some way closer to a state of nature (for a discussion of "raw" data, see Gitelman 2013). In the notion of "doing something with data," data production and collection is a preliminary phase in which one gathers data in order to use it toward some kind of insight gained through some kind of analytical processing (either at an end point or, more frequently, on a rolling basis). In QS, however, both the efficacy of tracking in drawing one's attention to details (as when Fabio told me that he realized he was spending more time on unimportant relationships that on the ones that mattered) and insights that result from the processing of data collected prior, are often glossed under a broader notion of "mindfulness."

Mindfulness was a dominant theme in the Bay Area QS Conference in the fall of 2012 and has been a minor yet very present theme in other events I have attended. In session after session, participants talked about the process of self-tracking as an exercise in drawing and focusing attention to particular areas of their lives. One of the presenters at the 2012 conference, Nancy Dougherty, demonstrated a light-up smile tracker that she had made. A sensor near her temple triggered an array of blue Christmas lights every time she smiled (see Dougherty 2013). The lights, she told the audience, made her realize how frequently she smiled throughout the day in various situations. Another presenter at the same conference discussed the way the practice of food tracking made him more mindful of nutrition, even without an explicit effort to implement a particular diet. Another QS participant told me about an experiment he was doing with a heart rate monitor that alerted him whenever his heart rate went over a certain number. The alerts, he said, were helping him to pinpoint the triggers for anxiety in his life by making him more aware of them as they happened. In these ways, self-tracking was cast by QS participants as a way of making certain kinds of behavior or phenomena more present for the tracker. This "making more present" most often meant noticing phenomena as they happened, "in the moment," as with Nancy Dougherty's Christmas lights, but was also sometimes understood in after-the-fact insights drawn from the data, as when Nancy, having removed the lights, continued to download the "smile count" collected by her sensor at the end of each day.

That the mindfulness that data bring to experience is of a specific kind was illuminated by a conversation I had when I took a walk one evening with a group of participants at the 2013 QS Conference in Amsterdam. A woman I will refer to here as Nicki (not her real name) told me that she had stopped tracking altogether over the previous year, though she remained active within the QS organization. She said she had stopped because she felt like she had become a "prisoner to the numbers." In its place she had taken up ecstatic dance. The contrast between tracking and ecstatic dance is revealing. Both might be understood as a practice of mindfulness and presence, but they operate very differently. Ecstatic dance is about losing oneself in the moment such that details become ephemeral: noticed, released, and forgotten. It invests deeply in experience as undifferentiated, uncapturable, and irreducible. In self-tracking, the mindfulness is one of attention to detail in which particular facets are pulled out of the ephemeral, fixed and recorded.

Nicki's shift from tracking to ecstatic dancing with its emphasis on ephemerality and undifferentiation also draws our attention to the relationship between fixedness and motion in photography, film, and data. If film is a series of fixed images viewed in rapid succession so that they appear to move in "real time," data are also frequently viewed as "in motion" over time and trackers often cite the movement of data (usually, though not always glossed as progress). Images, film, and data become fixed in time in ways that lend a sense of authority, or facticity, over the past where human senses and memories can be unstable, even untrustworthy. Yet unlike film, data-tracking projects are as often open ended; there is no end in sight for Michael's management of "that guy," for example. The ways in which data come to render a person, then, are always also, at least potentially, in a state of becoming. In this sense, then, data define and fix past experience in ways that are oriented toward data yet to come.

For the most part, the "yet to come" that data orient toward is not just more of the same, but a future that improves over time. While some mindfulness projects within QS, like Nancy Dougherty's, seem primarily curiosity driven, many more, if not most, tend toward addressing something in the tracker's life, whether an actual problem that presents challenges, a sense that something could be better, or just a general desire to "optimize." In this sense, self-tracking in the Quantified Self community has a definite bent toward self-improvement. In his introduction to QS, a volunteer leader at a meetup I attended in Portland, Oregon, in 2014 noted that QS has frequently been seen by detractors as navel gazing in which participants are absorbed by their selves as "special snowflakes." "We are," he said, "special snowflakes, but special snowflakes in the best possible way because we use our data and our projects toward becoming our better selves." Self-tracking data, then, hold out the promise of a capturable, knowable self that is also a manageable, and ultimately an optimizable self.

## Ninety-six Days Later

This chapter, more like film and less like a self-tracking project, has an end point that has taken shape slowly over the past three months and four days since I reread Benjamin's essay on "The Work of Art in the Age of Mechanical Reproduction" and wondered at the remarkable parallels between that discussion and the current moment. Working through these parallels has helped illuminate how self-tracking data construct and fix experience through the selection and recording of what is and is not counted, and how data "work" through proximity and distance to lend trackers a vantage point from which to view themselves and their experiences. I have argued that the commensurability of data works at a conceptual level that moves beyond the individual person and the idiosyncrasies of both the data projects and the data collection streams, and that in QS, these commensurabilities become organized into stories in which we both render and recognize ourselves in new ways.

For Benjamin, the transition at hand was from an art that vested its works with their own aura of specificity rooted in ritual and religion to an aura-less art available to manipulation in the politics of war, or (as in Baudrillard) the marketplace. In Benjamin, however, the subjects of capture (people, places, landscapes) are not particularly at issue. They remain largely the same. In the first half of the twentieth century, the technologies for capturing and the capacity for mass distribution were what shifted and turned representation into abstraction. In our own moment in history, capacities for duplicating and distributing data have likewise undergone rapid expansion to the point where the tiniest of devices can generate, process, and move data in volumes and at speeds that not so long ago would have taken a room full of processors to accomplish. In addition, the sheer proliferation of such devices over the past few decades is staggering. Yet unlike in Benjamin, I would argue the underlying mechanism of data as abstraction has not substantively changed. Data, to the extent that they are a representation of phenomena in the world through the marking, measuring, and tracking of some aspect or element of those phenomena, are always already an abstraction. What has shifted is not the operation (as Benjamin argues for artistic representation in film) but the objects to which we apply that process. It is not the fact of abstraction that is different in the twenty-first century, but the widening array of phenomena at ever-increasing scale and decreasing increments. It is the penetration of the kind of detailed capture in film that Benjamin describes as leading to the "cult of personality" applied to Everyman. What happens when we all become abstractions of ourselves is a question we have already begun to answer in the proliferation of selfies and self-rendering across social media sites. In tracking oneself, however, one begins to construct new kinds of significance, new kinds of specificity, from new kinds of details. We tell new kinds of stories, and we see ourselves in these stories in new kinds of ways.

Hélène Mialet, in her unpacking of an interview she had with Stephen Hawking, argues that the array of technologies and people that surround him surface the broader truth of the ways that self can be, and is in fact, distributed (Mialet 2003); we extend ourselves through our iPhones, our email, our avatars, and even sometimes, as with Hawking, through other people. What if the shift at hand is one of re-vestment? What if the proliferation of data and its penetration into daily life, as much as it abstracts our lives, is also a rearrangement of aura, and how it works? Certainly it is true that the ongoing tracking of our physical selves through such measurements as heartbeat and weight have revealed not only variations, but also uniqueness. What happens when specificity and abstraction collapse into one another? In a world of quantified self, here meaning not the organized meetups of the preceding discussion, but the broader term taken up by media and industry, perhaps we, like Hawking, extend ourselves through our technologies and our measurements and our recorded traces into our datasets, revesting them with something of our own selves.

The very notion of a "quantified self," while it retains the commensurability that lies at the heart of quantification, is here tied to a self, albeit one identified with an indefinite article: a self, not myself, or yourself. In the binding of quantification not merely to bodies or populations but with selves, data has taken on valences that move beyond the physical, material world, and into the ways we understand not only what we do, but who and what we are: ourselves. Lisa Gitelman, in her edited volume *Raw Data Is an Oxymoron*, points out that data "produce and are produced by operations of knowledge production" (2013, 3). In other words, she suggests that data produce and are produced by epistemologies. I am wondering if, in an age of accelerated data, data have come to produce and to be produced by ontologies: not merely ways of knowing, but also ways of being.

## Notes

1. A note on naming: several of the material resources I discuss here are drawn from or have been presented in talks given at various Quantified Self events and are posted on the Internet. In these cases, I have used the presenters' real names and links to their QS talks can be found under "works cited." In those cases where I draw on personal conversations and no public talk on the topic was given, I have followed anthropological tradition and used pseudonyms to protect the identities of these informants, though they may recognize themselves.

2. These latter details, not included in his notations but represented in my own field notes, arguably represent a different kind of "data" than that discussed in this chapter. This chapter is focused on data as it is discussed, practiced, and articulated within the QS community. I would argue, however, that the implicit understanding of what is and isn't data that is articulated through practices within QS is, in fact, largely representative of the ways data is understood and practiced in the general public: loosely, imprecisely, yet consistently as the capture

or recording of information that indexes an array of facts, feelings, activities, experiences, achievements, and events that, in the aggregate and through a set of often blackboxed analytics can, or should, lead to something called "insights." The extent to which anthropological data—generally recorded through a range of "scratch notes" and "field notes" and expressed through a range of rhetorical practices that Clifford Geertz famously captured as "Being There" (Geertz 1988; see also Sanjek 1990, and Clifford and Marcus 1986)—participates in the kinds of abstraction and commensurability discussed here is worthy of further discussion, though outside the scope of this chapter.

## References

Baudrillard, Jean. 1994. *Simulacra and Simulation*. Ann Arbor: The University of Michigan Press.

Benjamin, Walter. 1968. "The Work of Art in the Age of Mechanical Reproduction." In *Illuminations*, 217–251. New York: Schocken.

Clifford, James, and George E. Marcus. 1986. *Writing Culture: the Poetics and Politics of Ethnography*. Berkeley: University of California Press.

Cohn, Michael. 2014. http://quantifiedself.com/2014/04/michael-cohn-tracking-commitment/. Accessed August 31, 2015.

dos Santos, Fabio Ricardo. 2015. http://quantifiedself.com/2015/01/fabio-ricardo-dos-santos-using-relationship-data-navigate-chaotic-life/. Accessed August 31, 2015.

Dougherty, Nancy. 2013. http://justadandak.com/quantified-self-and-mindfulness-how-smiles-light-up-a-room/. Accessed August 31, 2015.

Geertz, Clifford. 1975. *The Interpretation of Cultures*. New York: Basic Books.

Geertz, Clifford. 1988. *Works and Lives: the Anthropologist as Author*. Stanford, CA: Stanford University Press.

Gitelman, Lisa. 2013. *Raw Data Is an Oxymoron*. Cambridge, MA, and London: MIT Press.

Mialet, Hélène. 2003. "Reading Hawking's Presence: An Interview with a Self-Effacing Man." *Critical Inquiry* 29:571–598.

Sanjek, Roger. 1990. *Fieldnotes: The Makings of Anthropology*. Ithaca, NY, and London: Cornell University Press.

# 3

# Biosensing: Tracking Persons

Sophie Day and Celia Lury

## Introduction

Biosensing is proliferating: sensors can be embedded in glaciers to monitor global warming, act as "labs on a chip" or as components in monitoring devices that function as a form of care. So-called self-sensing lifestyle devices attract excitement among consumers and industry alike and promise to enable us to bypass medical, financial, and other forms of authoritative knowledge production. Appeal is made to idioms of inclusion, DIY experimentation, and the redistribution of expertise, but, in parallel, contentious questions about privacy, ownership, and surveillance have emerged. How do such competing interpretations of the potential of biosensing coexist? In this chapter we introduce a range of examples to suggest that they are a response to, and can be understood best in terms of, the increasing importance of a particular organization of *observation* that supports practices of *tracking* in biosensing and in a wide range of other observational practices. We argue further that these practices recognize forms of personhood that challenge the political and legal construct of the person as individual.

In developing this argument, we make use of a very general sociological understanding of observation as "indicating something by means of distinction."[1] With this understanding, the collection of data *as* data can itself be seen as observation. If data are necessarily an observation, we could propose an understanding of tracking in terms of practices in which observation, or the collection of data, is folded—*looped*—into their analysis repeatedly and thus serially or recursively at defined intervals in time.[2] The recursive looping turns observations or traces made through data collection into tracks: it makes data meaningful insofar as the traces are related, linked, or connected to each other.

Our argument is that tracking is becoming an increasingly significant and diverse set of techniques in relation to the ongoing reconfiguration of relations between the observer and observed, and between observers. This reconfiguration includes not only the proliferation of individual sensing devices associated with a growing diversity of platforms, but also the emergence of new data infrastructures that pool, scale, and link data in ways that promote their repurposing (Kitchin 2014), opening them up to the use of analytics that produce a patterning of data as a dynamic problem space. It is in this space, so we suggest, that practices of tracking are coming to be implicated in new ways of making public-private distinctions that are themselves linked to changing forms of personhood and the reconfiguring of relations between market and state, economy and society.

We develop this argument in what follows through notes on contemporary examples of data use, a consideration of the public-private distinction, and a discussion of forms of tracking.

## "Personal" Data and the Private-Public Distinction

Our first example is the case of the incorporated woman. In what started as an art project, a person named Jennifer Lyn Morone has become a corporation: Jennifer Lyn Morone™ Inc (JLM). This project to establish the value of a person in a data-driven economy was initially a response to a brief that was part of a master's degree at the Royal College of Art, London, to "design a protest." The project highlights the appropriation of personal data by corporations through establishing provocatively a specific person as a corporation that "derives value from three sources, and legally protects and bestows rights upon the total output" of that person. The sources, reports[3] inform us, are: the accumulation, categorization, and evaluation of data generated as a result of Jennifer Lyn Morone's life; her experience and capabilities offered as biological, physical, and mental services; and the sale of her future potential in the form of shares. As a protest, this project thus draws attention to, and caricatures, that extraordinary legal fiction whereby the corporation is seen as a person and accorded the legal rights of natural citizens.[4]

As a development of the project, data from Jennifer Lyn Morone's life are to be captured and stored on the corporation's own servers, via a software application that will be known as Database of Me, or DOME. The goal is to create a software "platform" for personal-data management; companies and other entities will be able to purchase data from DOME via the platform, but their use of the data would be limited by encryption or data tagging. The software is thus to act as an automated data broker in a way that configures the person *as an individual*, that is, as a person whose agency is recognized in a relation to property established through the exercise of (self-) possession.[5] Indeed, having calculated that a substantial sum had been "invested" in her person over her life, Morone, as CEO, has also decided that JLM should offer: biological services, ranging from blood plasma at £30 ($50) and bone marrow donations ($5,100) to eggs at $170,000 apiece, and mental services such as problem solving (discounted if JLM gains something in return, such as knowledge), and is considering how to value services she currently gives away freely, such as compassion.

This project of incorporation is described as an experiment as well as a protest and an art project. Another experiment that gained publicity at the time we were writing was that conducted by Facebook during the week of January 11–18, 2012.[6] This study, published as "Experimental Evidence of Massive-Scale Emotional Contagion through Social Networks" (Kramer, Guillory, and Hancock 2014), sought to test whether "emotional contagion" occurs independently of in-person interaction between individuals by reducing the "amount of emotional content" in both positive and negative posts in the News Feed of Facebook. The authors described the conduct and reporting of the experiment as "consistent with Facebook's Data Use Policy," but the research was widely condemned as unethical. The ensuing debate led to an editorial entitled "Expression of Concern" by Inder M. Verma (2014), the editor in chief of *Proceedings of the National Academy of Sciences,* who described the best practice for obtaining informed consent and allowing participants to opt out; she notes that private companies, unlike public institutions, are not obliged to conform to this "Common Rule."

These two examples might be seen as inversions of each other. In the first, an individual tries to acquire for herself the economic value of personal activities by becoming a corporation and, in the second, it is a corporation that attempts to acquire and maximize value by collecting the traces of interpersonal activities. As such, they might be taken to indicate a deep fault line between private and public in practices of biosensing, where manipulating private emotions or bodily states for corporate profit causes ethical or moral concern. However, as our next pair of examples suggest, this line is not fixed or given but continually (re-)produced. In thinking about this continuous re-making, we have been inspired by Susan Gal (2002), who conceives the public-private distinction as the outcome of subdivisions, recalibrations, and fractal recursions. She writes:

> [W]hatever the local, historically specific content of the dichotomy, the distinction between public and private can be reproduced repeatedly by projecting it onto narrower contexts or broader ones. Or, it can be projected onto different social "objects"—activities, identities, institutions, spaces and interactions—that can be further categorized into private and public parts. Then, through recursivity, and recalibration, each of these parts can be recategorized again, by the same public/private distinction. (Gal 2002, 80)

Importantly, these distinctions do not all line up: as Gal notes, the definitions of public and private "are partially transformed with each indexical recalibration, while deceptively retaining the same label and the same co-constituting contrast." Following Gal (2002) we also suggest that the intertwined public-private pair is not a single division, but a recursive fractal.[7] Significantly Gal further argues that we often fail to see the public-private as a recursive fractal because "[o]nce named and thus semanticized, the fleeting distinctions of different roles, spaces and categories indexically invoked in interaction turn into 'reified objects' of the social world that seem solid and distinct" (2002, 85). Indeed Gal uses the notion of ideology to describe the categorization of public-private as a single division or dichotomy since it erases the dynamic recalibration of distinctions performed through the recursive use of indexical signs. The construct of the individual, we suggest, may also be seen in such ideological terms. However, while Gal suggests that indexical signs are typically ephemeral, we propose that they are increasingly widely supported in assorted data infrastructures, each of which has its own memory system. Indeed, we suggest, such developments may destabilize the ideological construct of the individual linked to the public-private distinction that has historically been such a dominant form of the person in many societies.

Consider, in this respect, our next pair of examples. A *Science* (Gymrek et al. 2013) article, "Identifying Personal Genomes by Surname Inference," suggests that genetic privacy is most likely impossible in the context of our cultural investment in ancestry. Melissa Gymrek et al. show that publicly available data, accessed through freely available Internet resources, allow you to infer the identity of "anonymous" genomes or sequencing datasets that are shared among scientists without identifiers. By profiling "short tandem repeats on the Y chromosome (Y-STRs) and querying recreational genetic genealogy databases," the authors recovered surname data that, in combination with other types of metadata such as age and state, enabled them to identity the "target."[8] Although the authors of this article do not themselves make public these links between the names of persons and genetic sequences, they offer the example of

Craig Venter, who was widely known to have sequenced his own genome. The authors show that the use of shared (public) family data or pedigrees enables an unidentified genome to be characterized as Venter's with reasonable certainty: "A search with Craig Venter's haplotype returned a clear match to a 'Venter' record that was concordant at all 33 comparable markers and with an estimated TMRCA of less than eight generations. … We further tested whether it would be feasible to trace back Craig Venter by combining the inferred surname with demographic profiling. A query for 'Surname: Venter; Year of Birth: 1946; State: California' in online public record search engines retrieved two matching records of males, one of whom was Craig Venter himself" (ibid., 323). In the same issue of *Science*, bioethicist Amy Gutmann notes, "A 'deidentified' genome has become a spectrum of possibilities for re-identification, rather than an absolute protection against privacy invasion" (2013, 1032).

The confirmation of these possibilities led a group of medical research bodies in the UK to accept the recommendations "that sanctions, such as the withdrawal of funding for or access to data resources, should be applied if researchers deliberately attempted to reidentify individuals from anonymized data. The group also set out the existing legal sanctions under the [UK] Data Protection Act, which include a maximum penalty of £500,000 for deliberately reidentifying participants from anonymised research data" (Wise 2014). Fundamental to such policies is a belief that trust will secure medical research for the public good. The report concludes with a citation from John Savill, chief executive of the Medical Research Council: "It's important that we protect the interests and anonymity of individuals while enabling research that benefits all of society. As funders we are committed to working together to reduce the risk of reidentification in a way that does not block valuable research to advance social and medical science and improve health" (ibid.).

The issue of trust—or its apparent obverse of trustlessness—has also been raised in relation to our fourth example of crypto-currencies, notably bitcoin (Mallard, Méadel, and Musiani 2014), for which the safety, integrity, and balance of its ledgers were, at least in its early days, maintained by a community of mutually distrustful parties referred to as miners.[9] These "private" currencies are seen by some to have the potential to provide an alternative to the national currencies of sovereign states, to undermine the ability of central banks to influence the price of credit for national economies, and to make it more difficult for national statistical agencies to gather data on economic activity for the benefit of the public.[10] At the same time, the "private" currency bitcoin also depends on an ideal type of public, in which trust is either irrelevant or taken for granted as part of the constitution of such a public. What is described as trustlessness derives from the transparency of the ledger, whose distributed, anonymized recursive operation on top of a P2P (peer-to-peer) network protocol[11] makes it difficult to fake transactions and generate anything resembling counterfeit currency.[12] As Mallard et al. put it, "every user that accepts to mine contributes a brick to the collective building of a trust that would, then, no longer need to be incarnated in specific institutional authorities." This second pair of examples thus suggests that the organization of trust(-less)ness—alongside (de-)individuation—also contributes to the making of the recursive fractals of the public-private.[13] There is no single distinction between public and private but multiple distinctions that do not all align: a private individual becomes a public entity through incorporation, but the resulting corporation addresses specifically the personal: a private currency has to be distinguished from a public one, but, in its mining or making, requires its own public.

To consider these fractals further we turn to our fifth case, which provides another instance of how the distinction between public/private is drawn, this time in relation to matters of security and (state) secrecy. We discuss this case in more detail to show something of the complexity of the production of the recursive fractal through forms of tracking that make use of repeated categorizations and calibrations. We then discuss tracking explicitly since we believe it is a set of observational practices that is coming to profoundly reconfigure the nature of the public-private distinction and to challenge existing forms of personhood.

## Tracking the Disappearing Plane

Our final example is the case of Malaysia Airlines (MA) Flight 370, the scheduled passenger flight from Kuala Lumpur to Beijing that lost contact with air traffic control on March 8, 2014 at 01:20 MYT (Malaysia Time), less than an hour after takeoff. The aircraft, a Boeing 777–299ER, was carrying twelve Malaysian crew and 227 passengers from fourteen nations. No crash site has yet been found and there has been no confirmation of any flight debris.[14] But how can a plane "disappear"? We suggest that "disappearance" is a consequence of a combination of "double blind" and "double bind" operating across what Luhmann (1998) calls first- and second-order observations. The former (first order) observes things; the latter (second order) observes things, including other observers, in their environment of observation. Any interpretation resulting from this second-order observation is, Luhmann says, likely to be both paradoxical and contingent.

To start our consideration of this case, we introduce some images. The first (figure 3.1) shows a ship falling off the edge of the (flat) world; this edge, or boundary, is redefined in the second (figure 3.2) as a horizon by hypothesizing a line of sight—of observation—between observer and observed in relation to a globe.

Our next image (figure 3.3) shows a diagram devised to track the possible movements of MA Flight 370 once it lost contact with air traffic control, that is, not only after the "seer" could no longer observe the observed but also after the observed stopped observing the observer, at least by the usual methods. In this image, we suggest, boundaries are drawn in the locally flat surface of a sphere.

To organize our analysis of these images we want to make use of a claim made by the artist Mel Bochner: namely, that boundary making is

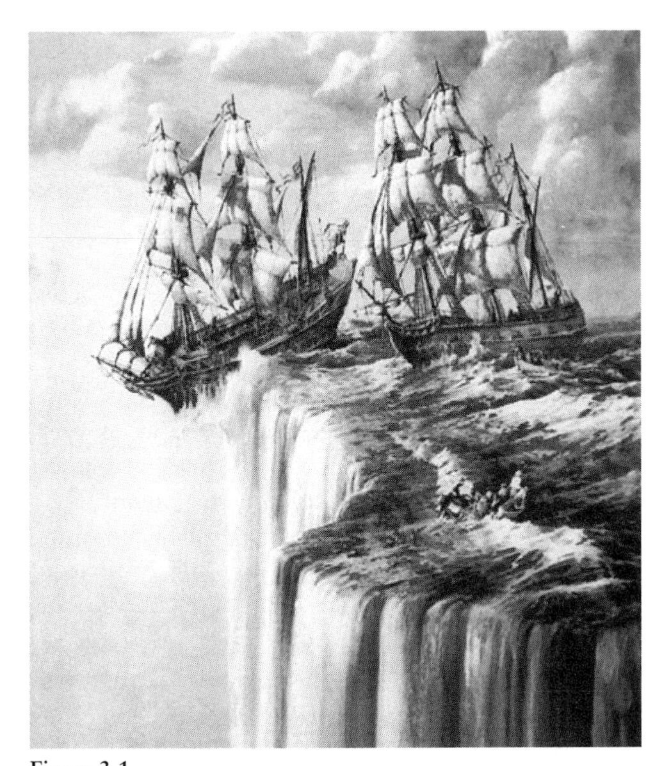

**Figure 3.1**
A late nineteenth-century map imagining how previous cartographers depicted a flat earth. Source unknown.

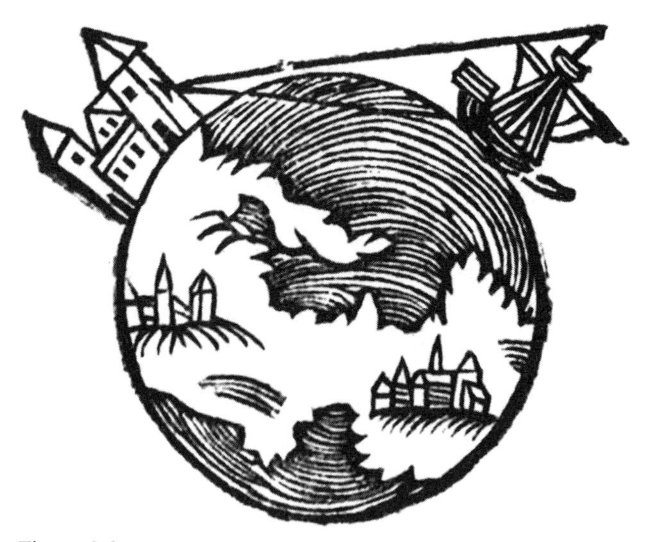

**Figure 3.2**
Picture from a 1550 edition of *De sphaera mundi* (On the Sphere of the World). Image in public domain.

"a hypothesis of sight," a process of composition (2008, 128). In relation to this last image, we suggest that the hypothesis takes place in relation to a surface of visualization, the organization of which produces a patterning of a problem space that configures what is visible and what is invisible, and indeed determines whether that invisibility or non-visibility is configured as secrecy, privacy, or, as in the case of MA Flight 370, disappearance. At a very general level, this organization is supported by a gamut of technical supports or platforms placed in specific relations to each other. Weber, for example, has shown how television emerges across the relations among three sites: the place of recording, the place of reception, and the place of transmission (Weber 1996). Increasingly, surfaces also emerge in the relations established among GPS, the military, governments, and everyday users of location-based devices and applications through algorithmic rules.

The initial hypothesis of sight that operates to produce boundaries in this case is, we suggest, what one of the founders of cybernetics, Heinz von Foerster (1995), describes as "double blind." A blind spot, or scotoma, is an obscuration of the visual field. A particular blind spot known as the physiological blind spot, or *punctum cecum*, is the place in the visual field that corresponds to the lack of light-detecting photoreceptor cells on the optic disc of the retina where the optic nerve passes. Since

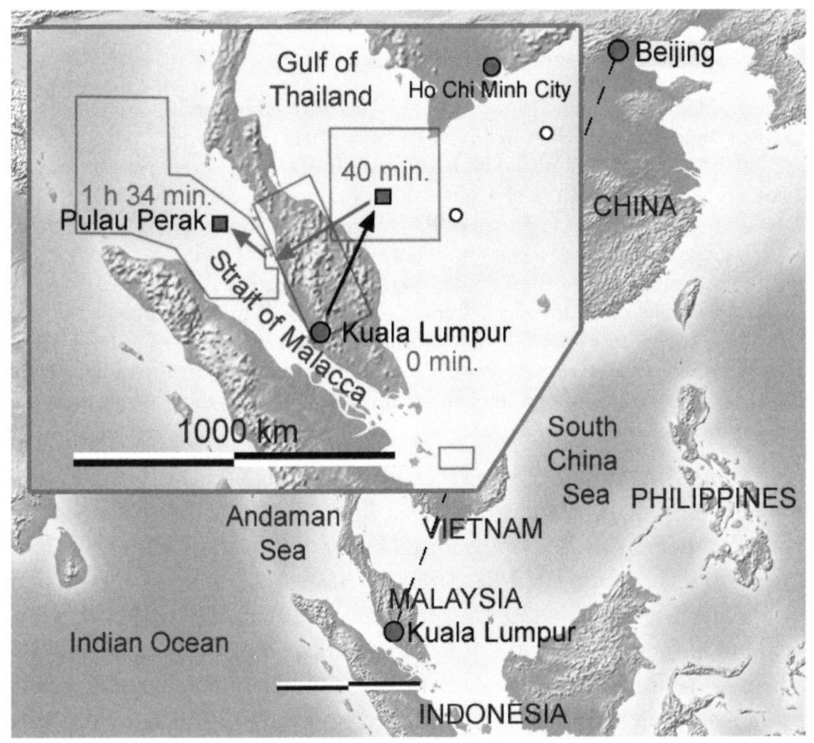


**Figure 3.3**
Route of Malaysia Airlines Flight 370 with search area inserted. Small circles indicate claimed debris sightings. Derived from File:Malaysia-Airlines-MH370_map.png and File:Malaysia-Airlines-MH370 search area.png. Wikipedia Commons.

there are no cells to detect light on the optic disc at this point, the brain interpolates surrounding detail and information from the other eye, with the result that the blind spot is not normally perceived. Interestingly, von Foerster does not discuss *the* blind spot but the *double blind*; indeed, he sums up the long-established finding that each of our two eyes has a blind spot with the aphorism: "We do not see what we do not see" (or as he put it elsewhere, "We do not see that we do not see"). And certainly, we live in an era defined by a cultural imaginary of total planetary observation made possible by the belief that, because of the multiplication of "eyes" to observe, "we" can see always and everywhere.

Laura Kurgan provides an example in her discussion of a sequence of views of the planet Earth that began with *The Blue Marble*, a photographic view of the Earth as seen by the Apollo 17 crew traveling toward the moon in 1972, and ends with analogous digital 2012 versions of this image. She describes these later versions as being

> ... assembled from data collected by the Visible/Infrared Imager Radiometer Suite (VIIRS) on the Suomi NPP satellite in six orbits over eight hours. These versions are not simply photographs taken by a person traveling in space with a camera. They are *composites* of massive quantities of remotely sensed data collected by satellite-borne sensors. ...This is not the integrating vision of a particular person standing in a particular place or even floating in space. It's an image of something no human could see with his or her own eye ... because it's a full 360-degree composite, made of data collected and assembled over time, wrapped around a wireframe sphere to produce a view of the Earth at a resolution of at least half a kilometer per pixel—and any continent can be chosen to be at the center of the image. [Moreover] ... it can always be updated with new data. (Kurgan 2013, 11–12; our emphasis)

*As a composite*, this image is especially interesting because it has no (visible) edges; that is, it appears to be a hypothesis of sight that does not make boundaries or, perhaps phrased better, is boundless. But, of course, the plane that disappeared has shown that "we" cannot see always and everywhere, even with the aid of the huge technical complex of GPS, civilian and military satellites, drone cameras, Google Maps, and so on. The disappearance thus reveals that there are edges (which might appear as gaps, corridors, out-of-focus patches, and the like) in the apparently boundless surface of visualization, even if we do not always know where they are or how they operate, where or when we might fall over these "edges."

This case of *double blind* is further complicated, however, by the operation of a *double bind*. The double bind is a phenomenon described by the anthropologist, fellow contributor to cybernetics, analyst of schizophrenia, and advocate of Alcoholics Anonymous[15] Gregory Bateson. Bateson suggests that the double bind—which he describes as "an experienced breach in the weave of contextual structure"—is a characteristic of all adaptive change. Such change, he says, depends upon feedback loops, "be it those provided by natural selection or those of individual reinforcement." He continues, "In all cases, then, there must be a process of trial and error and a mechanism of comparison." But, he notes, "trial and error must always involve error, and error is always biologically and/or psychically expensive. It follows therefore that adaptive change must always be hierarchic." The introduction of hierarchy is necessary since "[t]here is needed not only that first-order change which suits the immediate environmental (or physiological) demand but also second-order changes which will reduce the amount of trial and error needed to achieve the first-order change. And so on" (Bateson 1987, 201). Our suggestion, then, is that the disappearance of MA Flight 370 is a consequence of the emergence of a hierarchy of first- and second-order observation in the surface of visualization via feedback loops.

Let us explore this in a bit more detail. In the case of the disappearing plane, the *double bind* in operation for some, especially state actors, is the coexistence of the injunction to "see everything" (or at least the injunction, "do not see what you do not see") with the contradictory injunction to "see nothing" (which is to say, "do not see what you see"). The relatives of flight passengers in China and elsewhere most likely occupy a distinct position since they want to know what has happened to the plane and its passengers. They personify the imperative to see everything; they focus the minds of state actors who do not want to admit the failure of the fantasy of total planetary observation that is the *double blind* hypothesis. However in order for this double blind hypothesis to be preserved, observers who are differently situated in relation to the context(s) of observation would need to reveal to each other what they have (not) seen, and with this comes the challenging possibility of *comparison* of the capacity to observe. Comparison in turn has "costs" of very significant political tension for such observers, perhaps especially for observers acting on behalf of the state, intensifying the situation in which they simultaneously feel compelled to observe the injunction to not see what they do not see *and* to not see what they do see. These twin injunctions inform a slow dance of observe and (don't) tell, the outcome of which is both the creation and outcome of unstable hierarchies of first and second orders of observation, in which a plane can disappear, and in which mechanisms of comparison can only precariously establish what can and what cannot be seen.

And, not surprisingly, the disappearance of the plane was followed by a huge proliferation of hypotheses of sight, each of which reconfigured the distinction between security and secrecy. The actors or "eyes" who had an interest in, and the capacity to observe, the movement of the plane were many and various, including not only the Malaysian civil aviation department, air force, navy, and Maritime Enforcement Agency, but also numerous national and international bodies, resulting in the deployment of ships and aircraft from Australia, China, Japan, Malaysia, New Zealand, South Korea, the United Kingdom, and the United States. Significantly, for our interest in the hierarchy of first and second orders of observation, Wikipedia (a kind of composite eye itself) posted the following about "information sharing" among such actors/eyes:

> Although Malaysia's acting Transport Minister Hishammuddin Hussein, who is also the country's Defence Minister, denied the existence of problems between the participating countries, academics said that because of regional conflicts, there were genuine trust issues involved in co-operation and sharing intelligence, and that these were hampering the search. International relations experts said entrenched rivalries over sovereignty, security, intelligence, and national interests made meaningful multilateral co-operation very difficult. A Chinese academic made the observation that the parties were searching independently, thus it was not a multilateral search effort. ...
>
> Defence experts suggested that giving others access to radar information could be sensitive on a military level. As an example: "The rate at which they can take the picture can also reveal how good the radar system is." One suggested that some countries could already have had radar data on the aircraft but were reluctant to share any information that could potentially reveal their defence capabilities and compromise their own security. Similarly, submarines patrolling the South China Sea might have information in the event of a water impact, and sharing such information could reveal their locations and listening capabilities. (https://en.wikipedia.org/wiki/Malaysia_Airlines_Flight_370, accessed September 2014)

What unites the resulting multiple, competing, and variously credible hypotheses of sight that emerged to account for the problem of the disappearance of MA Flight 370 is, we suggest, the operation of various feedback loops between first and second orders of observation. Once double bind is in operation alongside double blind, not only may you not see what you do not see (the double *blind*), you may not see what you see, and you may also see what you do not see (the double *bind*), and so on. In the process, the feedback loops between first- and second-order observations produce "tracks" from "traces," which are, as Bateson says, "superposing and interconnecting." That is, the traces do not "make clear" or "lay bare," as in common usage, but result in a whole range of affective disorders of visualization—paranoia, narcissistic exceptionalism, and despair as well as the hope that the injunction "we do not see what we do not see" does in fact mean that we can see everything, and so can learn the fate of the disappearing plane and the people within it.

## Orders of Observation and Lines of Sight

So, what can "*we*" (the public?) observe in relation to this multiplication of "eyes" with which to see? Perhaps "we" can observe that the invisibility of the plane brings into visibility at least some of the technical supports necessary for observation, providing the possibility of piecing together knowledge about processes of composition in relation to, among other matters of concern, international security, secrecy, and the current technological capacity to observe in different media, including water.

We can begin to observe these processes from accounts that suggest the plane was first described as having disappeared when it crossed the edge of Malaysian and Vietnamese airspace, that civilian and military radar provided different information, that tracking via satellite could apparently provide information (technically speaking, "pings") about a change in direction but not whether this was to a northern or a southern corridor. Much less clearly visible, but still observable or rather observable by being rendered unobservable in specific ways, are the political dimensions that mean the information gained by both first- and second-order observation is only made available in particular ways by different actors. In short, what "we" can observe is that the plane's (possible) movements become variously visible (or invisible) in relation to different technologies of observation, mobility, and political and military "reach" (Allen and Cochrane 2010). What appears as a seamless, boundary-less 360-degree composite is shown instead to be a military-political-technical patchwork (figure 3.4), a ceaselessly ongoing collage with carefully stitched-together edges, corridors, and targets, international treaties, submerged alliances and territorial conflicts, satellites and submarines.

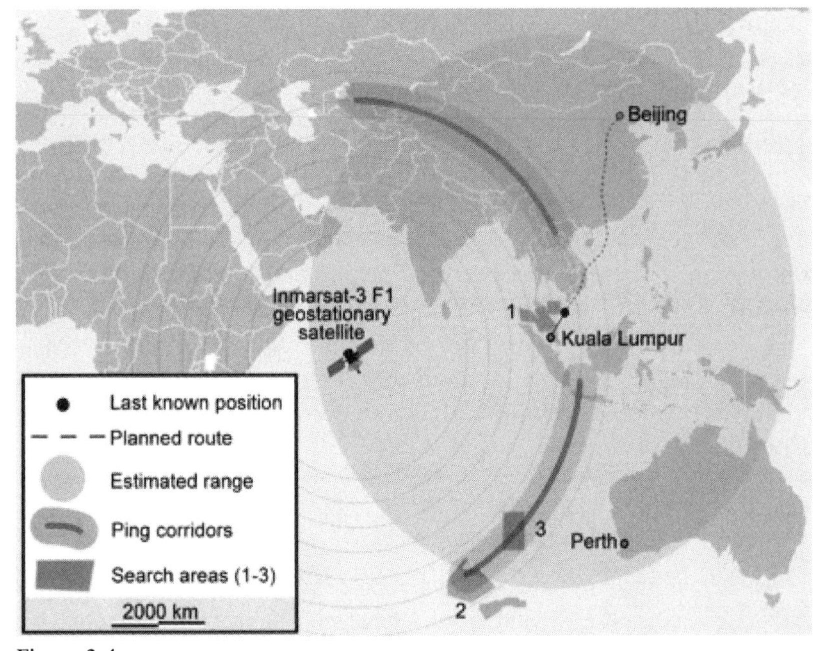


**Figure 3.4**
Map of search for Malaysia Airlines Flight 370 with search area inserted. Derived from Malaysia-Airlines-MH370_map.png and File:Malaysia-Airlines-MH370 search area.png. Wikipedia Commons.

To investigate the dynamics of this composition further, we can turn to discussion of other kinds of nonobservability, such as those of national state secrecy. Peter Galison, for example, points out that a targetable infrastructure has both come into view in recent years, and been rendered a matter of secrecy in the United States: "With the terror wars raging across the globe, sites previously invisible to the targeters—passenger trains, shopping centers, sports stadiums, monuments—suddenly came all too clearly into view" (Galison 2010, 962). And he suggests that it is "this targetable infrastructure" that informs the contemporary organization of state secrecy:

> After September 11, 2001, the whole system of national security began to shift, first with the Patriot Act (October 26, 2001) and then in a host of other alterations to the law. One key change in the secret universe was President George W. Bush's Executive Order 13292 of March 25, 2003. ... For Bush, the goal was to provide a system of information control that would continue the older "scientific, technological, or economic matters relating to the national security," but added to it the clause that this should "include defense against transnational terrorism" ... The government would seek as well protection to cover ... "vulnerabilities or capabilities of systems, installations, infrastructure, projects, plans, or protection services related to the national security, which includes defense against transnational terrorism." With this new vocabulary, especially in the inclusion of infrastructure, lay a sea change in the ontology of secrecy. (ibid) ... Bush framed the national strategy with a picture of the opposition: "The terrorist enemy that we face is highly determined, patient, *and adaptive*" (ibid, 964).

Galison concludes, "Our new security fence is everywhere, not delimited by time or space. ... Critical Unclassified Information fits our age exactly: a form of secrecy with no end date, no limit of scope, and little access through the Freedom of Information Act. In short we have a new ontology of hidden knowledge: multiply infinite secrets for a boundless conflict' (Galison 2010, 969–970). He suggests that the composite form identified by Kurgan allows for the multiplication of secrets, which in turn provide the grounds for conflict without end: not a composite of total planetary observation, but of infinite secrets for a total war (see also Chow 2006).

## Tracking: A Stitch in Time

How, then, are we to understand what is at stake for biosensing from this variety of examples? In what we have presented so far, we have added the notion of *composition* to Gal's conceptualization of the public-private distinction as a recursive fractal so as to draw attention to the specificity and variety of ways in which this fractal is now being produced. On the basis of our examples, we suggest that it is not simply the capacity to observe or sense that is being extended (that is, it is not simply the case that observers can observe more than before), but also the patterns of observation that are being complicated by these compositions. New practices of composition multiply the relations between observers, and in particular, the methods and kinds of feedback loops. And while we further suggest that many of these relations now commonly take the form of practices of *tracking*, we also note that their outcome is not pre-given.[16]

In a previous discussion of numbering practices (Day, Lury, and Wakeford 2014), we identified several processes of composition including zooming, folding, pausing, accreting, knotting, and diffracting. For example, we considered how fractions, including percentages, might be considered as practices of *folding* in which a denominator or whole is (recursively) folded (and unfolded) into (enumerated) parts. Here, in the discussion of the disappearing plane, we have suggested that such processes of composition can also be produced—via the use of feedback *loops*—as tracks. While the notion of a feedback loop was central to second-wave cybernetics, our examples indicate that it is now implicated in a variety of forms of tracking beyond what Hookway describes as the original "model space of a predator-prey relation" (2014, 107).[17] We suggest that this increasing *diversity* of forms of tracking (that is, not only but including hunting) depends on which hypotheses of sight are in operation, and whether and how levels of observation are introduced and how they operate.

To elaborate on both the importance and heterogeneity of tracking, we introduce an analogy with practices of stitching. The needle entering into the fabric being stitched indicates a moment of observation or data collection, the leaving of a trace, but this trace only becomes part of a track when a line is drawn, when a relation is established, between such points—in the case of stitching, by the thread that the movement of the needle leaves behind. It is this thread that is the track, and it is the effect of a dynamic process of composition, the stitching of the collection of data[18] across and between fabrics or spaces, running, edging, joining, hiding folds, superposing and interconnecting, all within the weave of the fabric or, as Bateson (1987) put it, the contextual structure that it comes to constitute.

One kind of tracking might be like a running stitch—the basic stitch in hand sewing and embroidery, on which all other forms of sewing are based (figure 3.5). The stitch is worked by passing the needle in and out of the fabric: a relation of observing the self by the self in a recursive observer-observed relationship, as with Jennifer Lee Morone Inc. In this case, the relation of separation between observer and observed that is essential for a trace to be recorded is effected by the incorporation of the person, a relation that, as we noted, acquires significance in terms of both the legal recognition of the corporation as a person and the history of the possessive individual. In this example, not only is the person as individual divided in herself by being incorporated, but her activities are also rendered as commodities.

Other kinds of tracking are more like blanket stitching (figure 3.6) in which an edge is secured: defining a territory or referent in relation to whose coordinates the object's movements are mapped. An example might be found in the mid-twentieth-century form of broadcasting where the "audience," in some sense observing television or other media, is constituted as a commodity to be bought and sold; the audience members' activities of watching in turn observed—or tracked—by broadcasters, who sell analyses of the traces of the individual or household activity of watching to advertisers. This is the count plus loop.

A third kind of tracking might be understood as invisible (or stealth) stitching, in which the detail if not the existence of a feedback loop between first- and second-order observation is hidden. EdgeRank,[19] the algorithm that Facebook developed to govern what is displayed—and how high—on an individual Facebook user's News Feed provides an example. The EdgeRank algorithm[20] calculated the sum of edges—where an edge was: "basically everything that 'happens' in Facebook. Examples of Edges would be *status updates, comments, likes,* and *shares*. There were many more Edges than the examples above—*any action that happens within Facebook is an Edge*" (emphasis in original). Each edge itself

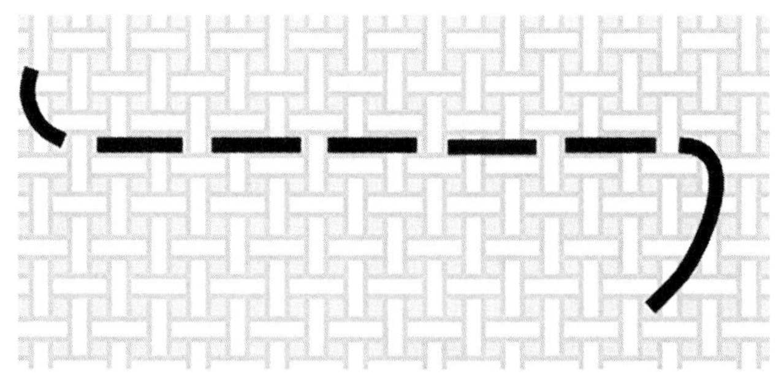

**Figure 3.5**
Running stitch. Public domain.

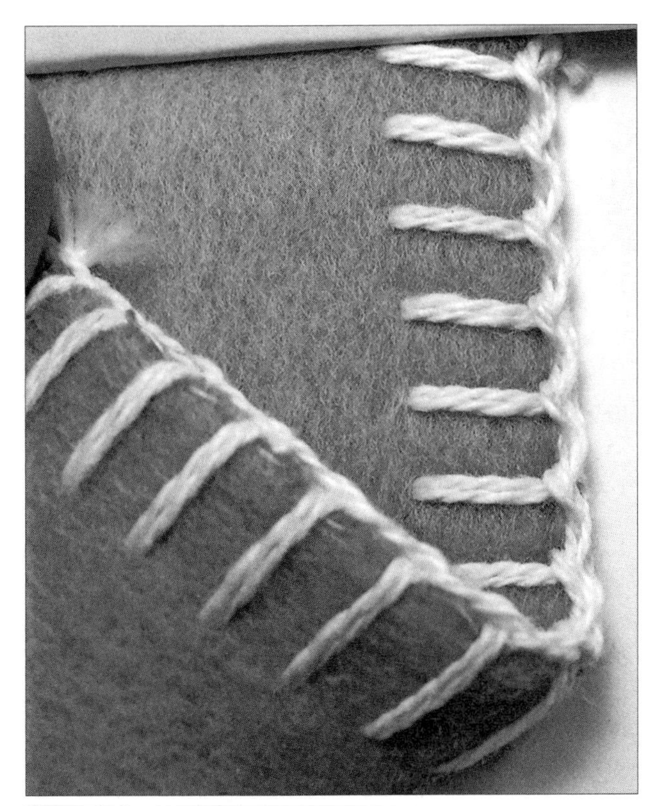

**Figure 3.6**
Blanket stitching. Wikipedia Commons.

was a composite of Affinity (a one-way relationship between a user and an edge), Weight (a valuing system created by Facebook to give greater weight to some actions rather than others), and Time Decay (Facebook's equation for this is 1/(time since action)).

In order for this stitching analogy to be useful, however, it is important to appreciate that the fabric in which the track is made visible is itself an ongoing contextual weave; as a consequence, tracking is constitutive and may produce knotting, fraying, or loose ends.[21] Indeed, to continue with the analogy, it was the existing operation of EdgeRank that made the Facebook experiment discussed earlier in this chapter appear uncontroversial to those conducting it: "Which content is shown or omitted in the News Feed is determined via a ranking algorithm that Facebook continually develops and tests in the interest of showing viewers the content they will find the most relevant and engaging. One such test is reported in this study: A test of whether posts with emotional content are more engaging" (Kramer, Guillory, and Hancock 2014).

In the light of other initiatives such as bitcoin, we suggest that likes, status updates, comments, and so forth can be understood as tokens in Facebook's own crypto-currency: they—and tokens in other proprietary social media—constitute transferable property rights in social connections, and specifically in dividuality (discussion follows). Indeed, Facebook might be seen to hold a monopoly in its own currencies, the value of which it can manipulate through continual recalibration of the rate of exchange.

## Conclusion: Tracking Persons

To conclude, we suggest that our examples do not simply support the claim that biosensing takes place in relation to a public-private distinction that is a recursive fractal, but indicate that this fractal is increasingly organized through a variety of processes of *tracking*, the recursive looping of data collection into data analysis. Not all loops are the same—tracks can be laid to make or seal edges, or to make invisible. Indeed, we have sought to show that tracking is central to the reconfiguration of economy and society, with implications for how we consider processes of securitization, financialization, and reterritorialization and deterritorialization whether performed as scoring, ranking, or edging.

In one further—more speculative—step, we return to the relation between the recursive fractal of the public-private and the longstanding legal and political fiction of the person. The developments in observing and tracking we have described here trouble this category of the person, which currently comprises both people and corporations. These ways of organizing observation track not an individual person that is undivided or persistently the same but, rather, a dividual, continually remade in relations that divide and connect.[22] Morone is parceled out, while Venter is reassembled through distributed datasets. We are not yet in a position to judge the outcome of this troubling of the category of person, but the issues at stake are suggested in some responses to the cases we have outlined.

For example, as we have indicated, crypto-currencies trouble the distinction of public-private. Indeed, we further observe that some currencies have adopted a playful approach to the project of personification by adopting a persona as a way of constituting—or masking—themselves as brands. But this strategy has met some resistance. For example, the currency Coinye initially used an image of rapper Kanye West as its logo. Upon hearing of this use, attorneys for Kanye West sent a cease and desist letter to the developers of Coinye, stating that the use of "Coinye" was willful trademark infringement, unfair competition, cyberpiracy and dilution, and instructing Coinye to stop using the likeness and name of Kanye West (Wikipedia, http://en.wikipedia.org/wiki/Coinye, accessed September 2014). In another example, the U.S. Internal Revenue Service has recently reasserted the construct of the person as individual by ruling that bitcoin would be treated as property for tax purposes and not as a currency. This move simultaneously made specific individuals identifiable for the purpose of charging capital gains tax (only individuals, not dividuals, hold property rights) and denied the legitimacy of the apparently im-personal guarantee provided by the distributed trustless platform for bitcoin as a currency.

Responses to the finding that it is possible to blur the distinction between a nonidentifiable and an anonymous person in relation to publicly available genetic data provide a further vantage point from which to view these developments. As we have indicated, commentaries on genomic sequencing variously query inconsistent state privacy protection, posit a continuum between public and private, and describe alternative approaches supporting open-access datasets and shifting norms of privacy. Sanjay Mehta et al., for example, advocate a "differential privacy" policy for related genomics problems, based on quantifiable thresholds to determine the level of aggregation of data open for analysis. As they note, "A new and different approach shifts the focus of privacy from being regarded as a property of the data, as reflected in the HIPAA de-identification standard, to account for the process by which information is disclosed independently of the data. The emerging standard in privacy protection and disclosure control, termed differential privacy, (…) is based on this approach" (Mehta, Vinterbo, and Little 2014). In the policy forum of *Science*, Rodriguez et al. refer to "an increasing number of 'citizen science' initiatives [such as Sage Bionetworks Commons and Genomera], which use informatics tools and social-media strategies to build research models for integrating participant preferences about privacy protection and future research use in an iterative and dynamic way" (2013, 276). In these proposals, it is implied that a person may now usefully be recognized—and given rights—not as an individual, but as a dividual, a form of personhood whose value(s) emerge in relations of division and connection, relations not of sameness but of self-similarity.

In short, the operation of recursion in all these examples, so integral to the expansion of forms of tracking we identify in this chapter, means that the edges of a person cannot easily be stabilized or secured. In consequence, relations to property *as* relations between persons constituted as individuals are in flux. It is too early to see clearly whether and how the legal fiction of the person (and corporation) as individual can withstand the challenge of experiments to capture the value of this emerging dynamic dividuality. But, in our view, it is this developing fiction that will (or will not) stabilize the recursive fractal of the public-private and provide the context for biosensing in the future.

## Acknowledgments

We would like to acknowledge Intel University Research Office, which supported our project on contemporary numbering practices (2011–2014) as part of a wider program on biosensors. This project supported our work with Nina Wakeford, whom we also want to thank. In addition, Sophie Day acknowledges research support from the School of Public Health, Imperial College London and the National Institute for Health Research Imperial BioMedical Research Centre, and Celia Lury acknowledges the support of the Economic and Social Research Council, grant no: ES/K010689/1.

## Notes

1. Luhmann defines observation as "any kind of operation that makes a distinction so as to designate one (but not the other) side. Such a definition is itself contingent, since what is defined would have another meaning given another distinction" (1998, 47).

2. This definition can be contrasted with practices of counting, one-off additive techniques in which analysis is separated analytically from the collection of data (see Day, Lury, and Wakeford 2014).

3. See P. H., "Who Owns Your Personal Data? The Incorporated Woman," *The Economist*, June 27, 2014, http://www.economist.com/node/21606113?fsrc=scn/tw/te/bl/theincorporatedwoman, accessed July 2014.

4. Among the many discussions of the corporation as a person, see Hart (2005).

5. The classic account of such "possessive individualism" is Macpherson (1962). While responses to the online article in which we first encountered this project suggest that the value of an individual's personal data might amount to no more than £10 a year, the magazine includes in its online report the observation that there are "13 trackers and beacons on this page alone."

6. As biosensing relies on social media platforms such as these, we do not make a hard distinction between such sensing and other ways of participating and knowing.

7. Gal's approach differs from Kelty's recursive publics (2005, 2008) insofar as she argues that the public is a derivative of the public-private coupling. Whereas Patterson and Nissenbaum (chapter 5, this volume) suggest that privacy is context dependent, our argument is that context dependence is actively produced as the specific process of patterning we describe here.

8. See Ana Gross (2015) for a discussion of the function "search" and processes of (de-)identification.

9. The more people mine bitcoin, the harder it is to generate. The situation now is such that the energy needed to mine requires more power than that of a typical household. Consequently KnCMiner (the company that used to sell bitcoin mining equipment) has recently built an industrial data center in northern Sweden in the Arctic Circle. From there, it generates bitcoin for itself as revenue, and leases power to customers; see http://www.coindesk.com/kncminer-cloud-mining-service-arctic-bitcoin-mine/, accessed September 2014.

10. They are not, however, seen by the Bank of England to "pose a material risk to monetary or financial stability in the United Kingdom" at present (All et al. 2014).

11. Mallard, Méadel, and Musiani (2014) provide a detailed description: "As a service operating on top of a peer-to-peer network, bitcoin allows users to execute payments by digitally signing their transactions. It prevents the possible problem of double-spending 'digital' coins through a distributed time-stamping service."

12. In the way in which it calls into question the legitimacy of the state's monopoly of currency, bitcoin evokes Simmel's (1950) discussion of the sociology of secrecy, where secrets index degrees of publicness in specific ways.

13. Mallard, Méadel, and Musiani (2014) write: "Bitcoin addresses—the virtual pseudonyms that identify users vis-à-vis the system—are the arrangement to which privacy protection for participants in the system is delegated. Each user possesses one or more bitcoin addresses that are stored and managed by its P2P client, its digital wallet. Each address is linked to a unique public/private key pair: … Bitcoin uses public-key cryptography, in which each user has a pair of cryptographic keys: a public encryption key and a private decryption key. The publicly available encrypting-key is widely distributed, while the private decrypting key is known only to its proprietor. The keys are related mathematically, but the parameters are chosen so that calculating the private key from the public key is either impossible or prohibitively expensive."

14. At the time of going to press, seventeen months after the plane disappeared, debris have been found washed up on Reunion that may yield evidence of a crash (BBC News, July 30, 2015).

15. Bateson (1987) claimed that his cybernetic epistemology coincided closely with the epistemology of Alcoholics Anonymous. Dawn Nafus pointed out to us that a parallel is commonly drawn between AA and the Quantified Self movement that has emerged in recent years.

16. As Bochner says, what is key to composition is not simply "the adjustment of the parts, i.e., their size, shape, color or placement to arrive at the finished work, but that the exact nature of that finished work 'is not known beforehand'" (2008, 37). See also Ingold (2007).

17. Hookway writes, "the teleology of cybernetics is an equilibration of behavior in the pursuit of a target, as a predator pursues prey. ... In this way, intelligent technologies evolve within the model space of a predator-prey relation" (2014, 107).

18. As Dawn Nafus observes (pers. comm.), engineers "stitch" together data that are qualitatively different—such as data referring to blood pressure and data referring to sleep. Combined, the stitches align the time stamps so that it is possible to see the joint trajectory of each data stream.

19. In 2011, Facebook stopped using the EdgeRank name internally to refer to its News Feed ranking algorithm.

20. This description of EdgeRank was taken from a webpage (December 2014) produced by Applum: http://www.whatisedgerank.com. Applum has produced a device called EdgeRank Checker that measures the average impact of EdgeRank; see http://applum.com. Other descriptions give alternative "formulas."

21. In discussion of these analogies, Dawn Nafus suggested that Facebook's poke feature might constitute an example of "fraying," used until so worn that it is cast aside.

22. We should note that we appreciate that persons relate "dividually" every day despite and alongside these norms (see, for example, Morris 1991). The concept of dividuality developed in Indian (Marriott 1976) and Melanesian (Strathern 1988) ethnographies has been greatly expanded since Marilyn Strathern's work deploying this perspective in Euro-American contexts.

23. The count (how many in the audience) plus loop (linking the counts together) defines the edge of the audience.

## References

All, Robleh, John Barrdear, Roger Clews, and James Southgate. 2014. "The Economies of Digital Currencies." Bank of England Quarterly Bulletin, Q3. http://www.bankofengland.co.uk/publications/Documents/quarterlybulletin/2014/qb14q3digitalcurrenciesbitcoin2.pdf. Accessed September 2014.

Allen, John, and Allan Cochrane. 2010. "Assemblages of State Power: Topological Shifts in the Organization of Government and Politics." *Antipode* 42 (5): 1071–1089.

Bateson, Gregory. 1987. *Steps to an Ecology of Mind*. San Francisco: Chandler.

Bochner, Mel. 2008. *Solar Systems & Rest Rooms. Writings and Interviews, 1965–2007*. Cambridge, MA: The MIT Press.

Chow, Rey. 2006. *The Age of the World Target: Self-referentiality in War, Theory and Comparative Work*. Durham, NC: Duke University Press.

Day, S., C. Lury, and N. Wakeford. 2014. "Number Ecologies, Numbers and Numbering Practices: Introduction." *Distinktion: Scandinavian Journal of Social Theory* 15 (2): 123–154.

Gal, Susan 2002. "A Semiotics of the Public/Private Distinction." *differences: A Journal of Feminist Cultural Studies* 13 (1): 77–95.

Galison, Peter. 2010. "Secrecy in Three Acts." *Social Research: An International Quarterly* 77 (3): 941–974.

Gross, Ana. 2015. "The Political Ontology and Economy of Data." PhD thesis. Centre for Interdisciplinary Methodologies, University of Warwick, Coventry, UK.

Gutmann, Amy. 2013. "Data Re-Identification: Prioritize Privacy." *Science* 339: 1032.

Gymrek, M., A. McGuire, D. Golan, E. Halperin, and Y. Erlich. 2013. "Identifying Personal Genomes by Surname Inference." *Science* 339: 321–324.

Hart, Keith. 2005. *The Hit Man's Dilemma: Or Business, Personal and Impersonal*. Chicago: Prickly Paradigm.

Hookway, Branden. 2014. *Interface*. Cambridge, MA: The MIT Press.

Ingold, Tim. 2007. *Lines: A Brief History*. London: Routledge.

Kelty, Christopher M. 2005. "Geeks, Social Imaginaries and Recursive Publics." *Cultural Anthropology* 20 (2): 185–214.

Kelty, Christopher. 2008. *Two Bits: The Cultural Significance of Free Software*. Durham, NC: Duke University Press.

Kitchin, Rob. 2014. *The Data Revolution*. London: Sage.

Kramer, Adam D. I., Jamie E. Guillory, and Jeffrey T. Hancock. 2014. "Experimental Evidence of Massive-Scale Emotional Contagion through Social networks." *Proceedings of the National Academy of Sciences of the United States of America* 111 (24): 8788–8790.

Kurgan, Laura. 2013. *Close Up at a Distance: Mapping, Technology and Politics*. Cambridge, MA, and London: The MIT Press.

Luhmann, Niklas. 1998. *Observations on Modernity*. Stanford, CA: Stanford University Press.

Macpherson, C. B. 1962. *The Political Theory of Possessive Individualism: Hobbes to Locke*. Oxford: Clarendon Press.

Mallard, A., C. Méadel, and F. Musiani. 2014. "The Paradoxes of Distributed Trust: Peer-to-Peer Architecture and User Confidence in Bitcoin." *Journal of Peer Production* 4. http://peerproduction.net/issues/issue-4-value-and-currency/peer-reviewed-articles/the-paradoxes-of-distributed-trust/. Accessed September 2014.

Marriott, McKim. 1976. "Hindu Transactions: Diversity Without Dualism." In *Transaction and Meaning: Directions in the Anthropology of Exchange and Symbolic Behavior*, ed. Bruce Kapferer, 109–142. Philadelphia: Institute for the Study of Human Issues.

Mehta, Sanjay, R., Staal A. Vinterbo, and Susan J. Little 2014. "Ensuring Privacy in the Study of Pathogen Genetics." *Lancet Infectious Diseases* 14 (8): 773–777.

Morris, Brian. 1991. *Western Conceptions of the Individual*. London: Berg.

P. H. 2014. "Who Owns Your Personal Data? The Incorporated Woman." *The Economist*, June 27. http://www.economist.com/node/21606113?fsrc=scn/tw/te/bl/theincorporatedwoman. Accessed July 2014.

Rodriguez, Laura L., Lisa D. Brooks, Judith H. Greenberg, and Eric D. Green. 2013. "The Complexities of Genomic Identifiability." *Science* 339: 275–276.

Simmel, Georg. 1950. *The Sociology of Georg Simmel*, trans., ed., and introduction by K. H. Wolff. Glencoe, IL: Free Press.

Strathern, Marilyn. 1988. *The Gender of the Gift: Problems with Women and Problems with Society in Melanesia*. Berkeley: University of California Press.

Verma, Inder M. 2014. "Editorial Expression of Concern." *Proceedings of the National Academy of Sciences of the United States of America* 111 (29). doi: http://www.pnas.org/content/111/29/10779.1.full.10.1073/pnas.1412469111.

von Foerster, Heinz. 1995. "Heinz von Forster [sic]." The Cybernetics Society. http://www.cybsoc.org/heinz.htm. Accessed September 2014.

Weber, Samuel. 1996. *Mass Mediauras: Form, Technics, Media*. Stanford University Press.

Wise, Jacqui. 2014. "UK Research Bodies Agree Steps to Protect Anonymity of Study Participants." *British Medical Journal* 348: g2372.

# 4

# The Quantified Self: Reverse Engineering

Gary Wolf

The Quantified Self is loosely organized affiliation of self-trackers and toolmakers who meet regularly to talk about what we are learning from our own data. I organized the first QS meeting with my friend Kevin Kelly in Pacifica, California, in October 2008. Today the Bay Area group has 4,193 members, and there are 110 other local groups. Last year there were about three hundred "Quantified Self Show&Tell" meetings around the world. If you'd attended one of these meetings, you would likely have seen between five and 150 people gathered in a classroom at a university, or the auditorium of a tech company or research center, showing tools and giving talks about self-tracking. In almost all of the events, the focus is on first person accounts of self-tracking projects. Speakers follow a simple format, typically answering these questions: "What did you do, how did you do it, and what did you learn?"

Many scholars participate. At our annual conferences in the United States and Europe, anthropologists, sociologists, and public health researchers often lead sessions that call upon self-trackers to critically examine their self-tracking practices. Meanwhile, self-trackers push back on the theoretical assumptions of the more academic speakers, drawing them into personal, pragmatic conversations about first-hand experiences tracking weight, exercise, food, sleep, symptoms of disease, or other experiences and measures. Many times, scholars at our Quantified Self meetings have joined in our particular style of reasoning, speaking in the first person and "for themselves." For instance Dawn Nafus, the editor of this volume, gave a talk in late 2013 about tracking her feelings after eating; Dana Greenfield, a medical student and PhD candidate currently writing her dissertation in the department of anthropology at the University of California, Berkeley (and author of chapter 7 in this book), opened our 2014 European meeting with an account of tracking her grief after the death of her mother; and Mark Drangsholt, a professor of medicine at the University of Washington, has given courageous talks about investigating his own heart rhythm disorder and an episode of cognitive decline.

In my response to the chapters in this part I'd like to repay this good faith by addressing an implicit question all the authors share: How can we talk about ourselves in the context of our self-tracking projects as if we were making consequential personal choices of our own free will when everything we bring into the conversation—tools, methods, interests, habits, and identity—bears the mark of what Adele E. Clarke and her colleagues have called "BiomedicalTechnoService Complex, Inc." BiomedicalTechnoService Complex, Inc. is a nickname that stands in for the powers shaping our experiences, choices, and potentials; more specifically, for the corporate and government domination of our minds and bodies. Just when we think we are taking our fate into our own hands, we're enacting rituals of obedience more effective in controlling us than external pressure, since they work from the inside. All the authors in part I work in the shadow of BTSC, Inc. even as they variously dispute its capacities. Mette Kragh-Furbo, Adrian Mackenzie, Maggie Mort, and Celia Roberts ask "Do biosensors biomedicalize?" They then go on to expose some of the dense forms of biosensing practice that twist and repurpose commercial and administrative tools on offer from standard suppliers. Sophie Day and Celia Lury wonder how idioms of inclusion and do-it-yourself experimentation can coexist with conflicts over privacy, ownership, and surveillance. They propose that these conflicts can't be understood when we take adjectives like "private," "public," "individual," and "corporate" as naming specific boundaries in our social world. Instead, we would do better to follow the linguistic anthropologist Susan Gal in understanding that "public" and "private" function as analogies, carrying the expectations we have about near things and far things across boundaries of scale, allowing us to think on our feet, although with a cost in conceptual steadiness and—importantly—a high risk of overconfidence in the sanctity of our supposedly personal life. Jamie Sherman notices that the self in a Quantified Self is often represented through numbers, graphs, and charts, and finds in this interest in factual detail something not merely illusory, but also sad, a feeling that she connects with nostalgia for an earlier era, when our personal experiences couldn't be captured by BiomedicalTechnoService machines.

Since all of these chapters are published in company with this one, my glancing descriptions aren't meant to give their arguments. But each of them shares a common belief: that the concept of the self has no simple coherence, except perhaps as part of a mythical past.

As Day and Lury write:

> In one further—more speculative—step, we return to the relation between the recursive fractal of the public-private and the longstanding legal and political fiction of the person. The developments in observing and tracking we have described here trouble this category of the person, which currently comprises both people and corporations. These ways of organizing observation track not an individual person that is undivided or persistently the same but, rather, a dividual, continually remade in relations that divide and connect. (chapter 3, this volume)

How strange, then, to notice that at Quantified Self meetings faith in the self is on full display. Week after week, we speak about ourselves as if we were born with Benjamin Franklin and schooled on John Locke. Although trackers describe projects explicitly designed to distance themselves from themselves, giving them a picture of their own experiences as if from afar, this is universally understood to be a kind of trick used by the presenter to awaken awareness, overcome the inertia of habit, and cast off illusion. Maneuvers of self-separation, carried out with varying degree of expertise, are unhesitatingly presented as techniques of enlightenment. Hasn't anybody noticed the trouble the self is in?

Many of the people who give these show&tell talks make money, more or less directly, from computing. They are engineers, designers, consultants, start-up founders. The meetings happen inside the offices of tech companies, consulting studios, and university classrooms associated with computer science and engineering departments. And those of us who don't work directly making hardware or software—the teachers, doctors, trainers, journalists, and so on—still typically have some kind of vocational stake in keeping current on tech trends. Normally, in these environments, people strictly look ahead.

In 2006, Genevieve Bell and Paul Dourish's paper "Yesterday's Tomorrows: Notes on Ubiquitous Computing's Dominant Vision," described a common trait of writing about the effects of having computing everywhere:

> The dominant tense of ubiquitous computing writing is what we might call the "proximate future." That is, motivations and frames are often written not merely in the future tense, describing events and settings to come, but describe a proximate future, one "just around the corner." The proximate future is invoked in observations that "Internet penetration will shortly reach ..." or "We are entering a period when ..." or "New technological opportunities are emerging that ..." or "Mobile phones are becoming the dominant form of ..."[1]

Although Bell and Dourish were addressing their colleagues (Bell is an anthropologist at Intel; Dourish a professor of informatics at UC Irvine), the mode of expression they described is widespread among future-makers in the environments where Quantified Self meetings are held, providing, as Adam Greenfield later wrote in his pamphlet "Against the Smart City," "an elegant way of dodging accountability for the frankly incredible assertions being made."[2]

So it's interesting to see at Quantified Self meetings how the future tense is deprecated. Instead of making speculative forays, we're going in reverse, poring over evidence, consulting dozens, hundreds, even thousands of observations gathered using every type of recording instrument, not just big data picked up by automatic sensors, but also photographs, penciled notes, once-a-day numerals representing a not-very-well-specified sense of well-being, sleep scores, step counts, place names, low blood sugar episodes. These backward-looking habits, organized around things that have their main significance only for the person who gathers them, resemble the compulsions of collecting. Instead of stamps, books, botanical specimens, or beer mugs, the self-tracker has numbers and numerical pictures whose style, however formal it may be, can't at all cover up their motley origin and history. The force that unites these materials is the force of possession: they belong together because "they're mine." And how much we do treasure these observations, across the whole span of their significance from trivial to astonishing.

"Perhaps it's the hoarding urge that drives so many of the Quantified Self initiatives," writes the critic Evgeny Morozov, decrying these projects of self-knowing as puerile and unaccountable:

> Of all the things to be hoarded, data—especially data stored in the cloud rather than on hard drives in one's bedroom—has all the right attributes. It doesn't take much space, it's easy to move, and if you play your cards right, you can even make some money off it. Small, mobile, lucrative: it's a perfect hoarding target for our hypercapitalist age. It is a perfect response to the riddles and anxieties of our complex times. … The problem is that, as firm, scientific data, [its] results have no standing. As moral prompts to action or conclusions drawn from months of self-reflection, they hold no standing either. … As the never-ending arguments over climate change show, we are already living through a period when trust in expertise is all but gone. Supplying those who want to challenge it further with odd theories of knowledge will only make things worse. … [T]he sooner we acknowledge this, the healthier our public debate will be.[3]

Leaving aside the question of whether expert authority needs the defense he mounts on its behalf, Morozov's polemic—and especially his reference to hoarding—usefully exposes a usually hidden reaction of disgust at practices that take official, industrial, standardized, known elements of our highly technologized world and use them for unsanctioned, deeply personal, and—from the outside—illegible reasons. If the self begins with sensations at the surface of the body and its openings, then new vulnerabilities attached to technology might easily provoke disgust, especially when they're revealed as abnormal.

Day and Lury catalogue trouble for individuals presumed to be persistently the same. The personal reasons offered by self-trackers for undertaking a self-tracking project often show an acute alertness to these troubles. Illness, for instance, rattles the self, especially when medical expertise fails and treatments don't work, or, worse, when even a diagnosis is lacking. Meanwhile, emotions control us as if from outside, and damaging habits stand strong against efforts to shake them. Although these challenges to self confidence are nearly as old as the moon, there's a special flavor here, because these threats to the self are visible against a background of smart machines, of drones, whose explicit branding of convenience and violence delivers an implicit payload in the form of a question: what if you yourself are a drone, programmed for action in a code you've never bothered to read?

The very first electronic life-logging device, a radio-signal-transmitting personal beacon, was made by its inventor Robert Gable to help juvenile offenders improve their self-control through positive feedback, reducing the probability of punishment. But the utopian promise of this and subsequent behaviorist interventions got tangled in the contradictions of its premise. There is no distinct class of experiences identifiable as "behaviors" except in relation to the rewards and punishments that sanction them. To maintain a link between action and consequence reliable enough for behavioral measurement requires stripping away the possibilities of accident, and cutting back on degrees of freedom using techniques of the lab, the casino, and the prison. I've been on a trip with Professor Gable to visit the offices where court-ordered ankle bracelets are placed on his unwilling legatees, and watched him think hard about what's gone wrong. Gable came up with his radio-tracker in the 1960s, and it took decades for its full toxicity to emerge. But if change is accelerating exponentially, then perhaps we've reached a point when the effects of the tomorrows we're making spill across a threshold into the present, crowding us in a way that makes everything appear foreign, including ourselves.

Whether the use case is travel security, accounting forensics, or medical compliance, nearly all systems of modern crowd control rely on techniques of personalization. The result of such detailed, multifaceted, administrative biography is to dissolve every person into a crowd of one, a jumble of traits knowable only in the aggregate, from outside. But when a self-tracker reaches into this ever present resource and seizes hold of some details, exposing a grab-bag of numerical observations now charged by the force of possession into mementos worthy of care, this has something of the weird effect you see when workers who are banned from striking decide to follow every rule. Things slow down. "We generally think of hoarding as pathology, but I feel that it is often an attempt at re-rooting, at halting the supersonic trajectory of modern cultures, at building a coherent nest in a windy world," said archivist Rick Prelinger, beautifully, last month.[4] Against BiomedicalTechnoService Complex, Inc, the Quantified Self counters with an imitation game, matching—in a kind of handcrafted forgery, and of course at an infinitely slower pace—both internal machines of biology and psychology and external machines of administration and surveillance.

Self-trackers look in two directions at once, dropping reminders along the way in anticipation of returning, like Hansel with his crumbs. As artifacts, collections face backward, but as an activity, collecting is acquisitive and speculative, encompassing the future. Such investments are hazardous, and in a sense disreputable. A claim to reach into the future with intention and to preserve the past in memory will strike demystifying critics as the most indulgent of fictions. How much hope can we permit ourselves that the future will be habitable; not merely habitable to life but habitable to *us*? What chance is there that we can return to a future that resembles, and in which we resemble, what we've dreamed of ourselves in the past?

## Notes

1. Bell, Genevieve, and Paul Dourish, "Yesterday's Tomorrows: Notes on Ubiquitous Computing's Dominant Vision," *Personal and Ubiquitous Computing* 11.2 (2007): 133–143.

2. Adam Greenfield, "Against the Smart City" (New York: Do Projects, 2013).

3. Evgeny Morozov, *To Save Everything, Click Here: The Folly of Technological Solutionism* (New York: Perseus Books, 2013), 232.

4. Rick Prelinger, Keynote Presentation, Personal Digital Archiving Conference, April 24–26, 2015, New York, http://www.slideshare.net/footage/personal-digital-archiving-2015-keynote-talk-by-howard-besser-rick-prelinger, accessed August 31, 2015.

# II

# Institutional Arrangements

Part II examines the institutions that have a stake in biosensors and biosensor data. As noted in the introduction, biosensors have been an important part of medical devices for many years, and only more recently have been sold directly to individuals. This shift in how devices are sold has implications for markets, medicine, and public policy. Medical institutions, device manufacturers, patient advocacy groups, scientific researchers, employers, and privacy advocates all seek a say in how biosensor datasets are used, who can use them, and who possesses the legal, scientific, or moral authority to interpret them. Much of this tussle is about control and power among institutions, while other aspects have to do with challenges over what is and is not subject to institutional control.

Each chapter examines a particular node of biosensing practice, where sensors or their data encounter institutional practice. For example, in Fiore-Gartland and Neff's chapter 6, the business discourse of "disruption" mediates the relationship between the technology industry that sells sensors direct to consumers, and the health-care industry that considers some of this data to be matters of clinical practice. In Greenfield's chapter 7, "n of 1" experimentation is a way that self-trackers describe what they do. This framing as a research-like practice opens up questions about the intersection of medical research practices, citizen science, and the nonresearch side of self-tracking. In chapter 5 Nissenbaum and Patterson look at information flows as a key intersection of technology design, social norms, and privacy law. Mehta, having been a technology startup founder, in chapter 8 looks at some of the practical aspects of managing the tensions within these intersections.

The chapters of part II show that biosensors intersect with institutions in a context where biomedicalization has already been thorough. We find no clearer example than Mehta's chapter, which shows how biomedical control is informally asserted over practices and technologies that are patently nonmedical in nature. In Fiore-Gartland and Neff's contribution, we find contested claims over what constitutes medical practice, and is therefore subject to medical regulation. While this contest is regulatory, it is made possible by more widespread biomedicalization, which medicalizes what is outside clinical practice. If "health" is everywhere already, then companies can argue that their data are for "informational purposes only," while also persuading their customers that having this information could improve their health. Biomedicalization also appears to have paved the way for self-tracking as a kind of counter conduct, which Greenfield compares to the appropriation of reproductive technologies by second wave feminists. These two situations have very different relationships to biomedicalization, however. "Disrupting" health care by shifting control to technology companies only displaces the actors but otherwise does not change biomedicalization, while appropriating the tools that biomedicalization has produced creates space for a more diverse epistemic culture.

Part II also makes clear that these exchanges between different types of institutions quickly become legal matters, whether in the form of privacy law, labor law, or laws governing medical practice. A difficult set of questions emerges about the circumstances in which legal solutions are more effective than design solutions, and vice versa. That is, where data go could be decided by law, or by how technology builders build the "pipes," or a combination of both. Mehta's work suggests that legal solutions alleviate the need for technology developers to put themselves at a commercial disadvantage by devoting resources to privacy management systems when competitors might devote their resources to gaining more customers. In this sense, the law levels the field of competition. But which set of laws, or regulatory bodies? Nissenbaum and Patterson's example of employers implicitly or explicitly coercing employees to collect continuous health, wellness, and lifestyle data, and report it back to the employer, suggests that labor law could be involved alongside laws governing privacy and medical practice.

Nissenbaum and Patterson provide a helpful way of examining how culture, institutions, and the law intersect. Where they emphasize norms and consensus concerning prevailing values, Greenfield describes a setting where values are not, in fact, shared. To my mind, seeing both of these cases side by side is incredibly useful, as it helps us distinguish where we do and do not have shared values. Being clear about instances where values are shared or contested can inform decisions about what is better handled by policy versus design. Where there is no consensus, or a false consensus, the law may in fact be the better venue. For example, in the employer-employee scenario Nissenbaum and Patterson describe, it seems implausible that a biosensing company that would sell health and lifestyle data to employers could also be trusted to act as auditors of information flows in ways that would protect employees. If those auditors share the values of the managers they intend to sell to, and take those values to be uncontested norms, employee problems that stem from differing views of these norms will be treated as nonproblems by the audit. The far-reaching normativity of the "good employee" that makes this business model conceivable cannot be openly contested by auditors, lest those auditors also be revealed to hold non-normative values. It might be too much to ask of people doing auditing work to stand up to this normativity without support from elsewhere.

This situation reminds me of Goffman's famous description of the "unblushing American," the rare creature with nothing to hide, who in practice could only be "a young, married, white, urban, northern, heterosexual, Protestant father of college education, fully employed, of good complexion, weight, and height, and a recent record in sports" (2009 [1963], 128). Such people are rare, but when power is in play, they become the standard against which the rest of us are measured. Data collection has historically served as a way of consolidating cultural and economic power. When unblushing objections cannot be openly registered, it seems that only the law can provide a check on the power data collectors have over data subjects. Most of us, in one way or another, will find ourselves on the wrong side of employers' gaze, and come up short. Who among us can declare ourselves to be anything but the unblushing American without incurring economic penalty?

This discussion of privacy recalls part I's theoretical contributions concerning how data are caught up in distinctions between self and other. Part II observes how these distinctions work in institutional contexts, where the dominant modern institutional form is the bureaucracy. Bureaucracies emphasize the impersonal and the rule-based, which intensifies the difference between self and other. They are designed to disembed organizations from the social relations they are in. It is no wonder that privacy recurs as a theme when bureaucratic organizational forms dominate the production of both technology and health care. They make self and other grow wider apart, and privacy violations become more likely.

More recently, bureaucracies have developed a tendency toward organizing themselves around audit (Strathern 2000). Audit cultures make people more responsive to the measures that institutions create, and thus less responsive to the people they are supposed to serve, who invariably have needs more diverse and less quantifiable than audits presume. It is undeniable that audit is one of the few tools at our disposal to create transparency when dealing with such organizations. It is also undeniable that transparency is sorely lacking when it comes to data flows. Without transparency it is all but impossible for people to object to the harms that come through poor data handling. At the same time, locating deliberations about privacy handling in audit practices could create more disregard for data subjects than attention and care. As Strathern observes, meaningful representations of context rarely fare well in audits, which are ultimately about institutional needs. Bureaucratically driven organizations could easily use privacy audits as an exercise in what could be called "privacy washing," and deliver less privacy protection rather than more. Perhaps measures to somehow close the social distance that creates privacy problems in the first place, like diversifying the kinds of institutions that handle data, are equally necessary.

Finally, part II gives an indication of the kinds of roles that individual biosensor users might play in relation to the institutions they must deal with. Mehta argues that the public would be better served if technology producers addressed people as consumers, not as patients. From the point of view of a startup founder, it is reasonable to see this as an either/or choice. However, many readers who are not in that position will insist that conceptualizing people as either patients or consumers is far too narrow, and leaves no room for state involvement. Civic advocacy is also an important role to play with respect to many institutions, including the state. Citizenship implies a broader set of shared interests than does patienthood or consumption. Indeed, the many people who find it offensive that health care even has "business models" would ask whether there are groups putting pressure on the state or other public-interest entities to assert privacy rights, rights to data access, or other matters.

Citizen-based advocacy is indeed a part of the biosensing world. In Greenfield's work, there is evidence of a growing patient movement advocating for better access to medical data. The "give me my DAM data" movement does vocally register complaints about lack of access to data with the U.S. Department of Health and Human Services, though these activists face well-resourced, well-connected adversaries. Perhaps uncoincidentally, at the time of writing there is proposed legislation to make it easier for health-care companies to reject requests for medical records, and to charge unlimited fees for accepting requests. This makes me wonder whether the problem patient advocates are trying to address can be solved from the position of patienthood *alone*. Could it be that more of us have not joined their fight to "give me my DAM data" because we do not yet see ourselves as "patients"? By the time we do become patients, it could be too late.

As significant as these efforts are, lobbying policymakers is not the only form of politics possible. The personal is indeed political, and the counter-practices that challenge the dominant, biomedicalizing model of what data are for can also make alternatives possible. These practices derive their political effectiveness from being the change they seek, and they may ultimately have the final word on what biosensing will be about. As the business gurus like to say, in the end culture eats strategy for breakfast. Taking cultural politics seriously does not mean that institutional forms can be ignored, however. Regardless of how a discipline theorizes institutions—and here we must recognize great differences in sociological, anthropological, and other approaches—it is impossible to have a discussion about things like the quantified self, or data cultures, without them.

## References

Goffman, Erving. 2009 [1963]. *Stigma: Notes on the Management of Spoiled Identity*. New York: Simon and Schuster.

Strathern, Marilyn, ed. 2000. *Audit Cultures: Anthropological Studies in Accountability, Ethics, and the Academy*. London: Routledge.

# 5

# Biosensing in Context: Health Privacy in a Connected World

Helen Nissenbaum and Heather Patterson

## Introduction

Socio-technical systems that enable communication between "smart" networked devices create a suite of new vulnerabilities for individual users and for society, the precise character of which reflect differences between entrenched and novel social practices. Here we argue that these vulnerabilities implicate privacy by virtue of disrupting settled information flows, and thus warrant a thoughtful consideration of the ends, purposes, and values of the underlying context in which novel information flows occur.[1]

Recent years have seen the emergence of a vast array of personalized self-monitoring tools, the use of which challenges long-entrenched social norms governing personal information sharing. Self-monitoring practices that began with sports and fitness bands and portable medical devices have rapidly expanded into new realms, facilitating caretaking of self and others and forging new inroads into health, wellness, and productivity from cradle to grave. Although these tools present exciting opportunities for raising awareness, building community, and improving efficiency and productivity, they also highlight tensions that animate contemporary privacy debates as individuals and societies discover, adjust to, and resist opportunities afforded by new technologies. A consideration of the precise nature of disruptions introduced by self-tracking technologies will help us determine whether new practices are problematic, and, if so, whether those problems are best approached with an eye toward legislative, policy, or technological solutions.

In this chapter we assess contemporary health self-tracking practices through the lens of Contextual Integrity, an analytical privacy framework that demands a full consideration of the social settings in which novel practices are situated, including the type of information at issue, the identity of the information subjects, senders, and recipients, and the social norms underlying the context in which new information flows occur. Our approach entails first a description of a novel practice, and second, a normative evaluation of this practice in terms of individual interests, social values, and contextual ends, goals, and purposes. We conclude with an examination of tools at our disposal to bring these systems in line with normative values, including law, policy, and technical design.

## A Taxonomy of Health Self-Tracking

To clarify our domain and anticipate terminological ambiguities, we first situate our argument and cases within the larger landscape of health self-tracking. As explained in this book's introduction, the class of health biosensor systems includes great variation in its instances, and along with this, great variation in the terms applied to them. Fitness bands, medical sensors, health apps, smart garments, workplace performance trackers, and home life automation technologies allow for the monitoring of a wide variety of bodily metrics across the lifespan of their wearers and within numerous social contexts. In observing the range of these systems, including their served populations, composition, and aims, we identified several factors that distinguish them:

- *System components* (e.g., hardware, software, and linked services for users and third parties);
- *Device form factors* (e.g., freestanding consoles in the home, wearable clothing and jewelry, patches and tattoos, and implantable or ingestible medical devices);
- *Input modalities* (e.g., automatic sensing, manual self-reporting);
- *Sensor capabilities* (e.g., accelerometers, weight scales, and respirometers);
- *Information types collected* (e.g., distance walked, body mass index, and respiration rate);
- *Aims of the system* (e.g., increasing awareness, deepening self-understanding, building community, automating or facilitating caregiving, enhancing workplace productivity, or managing insurance costs);
- *Actors in the circuits of information flow,* including *Initiators* (e.g., self, care givers), *Data subjects* (e.g., self, children, employees, patients), and *Data recipients* (e.g., self, online or offline friends, family members, colleagues, third-party wellness administrators, human resources personnel, insurance company officers, physicians, public health officials).

Delineating these factors provides axes of systematic differentiation among this burgeoning array of devices and services and helps distinguish between instances on which we focus in this chapter. Ultimately, this will be useful in teasing apart diverse systems and surrounding practices that are relevant to privacy.

## Health Self-Tracking and Privacy

At first glance, privacy would seem irrelevant to the domain of self-tracking—tracking *of* one's self *by* one's self. Other normative problems may come to mind: perhaps obsessive perfectionism or intense self-focus—but why privacy? The brief answer is that most self-tracking systems radically interrupt and divert preexisting information flows. According to the definition of *privacy as Contextual Integrity* that we adopt in this chapter, privacy requires the appropriate flow of information, which means flow that meets legitimate expectations. Legitimate expectations, in turn, are characterized by context-specific norms of information flow that not only are entrenched in the practices and conventions of a given context (for example, health care, education, religious practice, etc.), but that also support important ethical and contextual values.

If nothing else, these new technologies disrupt entrenched information flows by virtue of many of the properties we have noted already—namely, close and continuous monitoring of personal information through networked sensory apparatus and self-reporting, and the accumulation and use of this information not only by the data subject, but also by third parties. Additionally, the fact that many trackers are small and unobtrusive encourages ubiquitous wear, and their sensor capabilities and flexible input modalities allow the logging of a full complement of detailed user behaviors, such as when individuals wake, bathe, eat, work, recreate, and sleep. Commonly branded as tools for healthful and positive lifestyles, they tacitly encourage honest and complete engagement. Yet the ecosystem within which these trackers actually function, including interoperable "smart" devices, apps, and services facilitating third-party access to information that may be collected, distributed, assembled, and mined, belies the user's subjective experience of a truly closed system of self-tracking.

These constitute the prima facie infringement of existing informational norms due to radical alterations of the type, frequency, breadth, and depth of information tracked, how it is tracked, and who has access to it. These observations do not answer the question of whether self-tracking systems violate privacy. They merely indicate why we need to ask the question of whether disruptions are appropriate.

**Contextual Integrity**

According to the framework of Contextual Integrity, what people care about is not that we should have complete control over information about ourselves, or that no information about us should be shared, but that it should be shared appropriately (Nissenbaum 2009). Contextual Integrity is predicated on the notion that social contexts are an organizing principle of social life, in that people do not act or transact merely as individuals in an undifferentiated social world, but rather as actors, operating in "structured social settings characterized by canonical activities, roles, relationships, norms (or rules), and internal values (goals, ends, purposes)." Context-dependent informational norms embody appropriate information flows by prescribing (and proscribing) what types of information, and about whom, may be transmitted by whom and to whom, and under what constraints. Thus the framework posits the parameters of *actors* (subject, sender, and recipient), *information types*, and *transmission principles*, each ranging over the ontologies that constitute respective social contexts. When actions or practices violate entrenched informational norms, they provoke protest, indignation, or resistance. When actions or practices are in compliance, they respect contextual integrity.

More widely, information technology and digital media have aroused deep concerns over privacy, according to this theory, because they are responsible for massive disruptions in the ways information (or data) *flows*—ways in which it is captured, utilized, and disseminated. Before we can begin to evaluate whether these disruptions should be welcomed or resisted we must clearly understand their nature and sources. Contextual Integrity offers a way to do both—to locate and describe disruptive flows and also to guide assessment in moral terms. A heuristic emerging from the theory suggests key steps: (1) establish a prevailing *context* for the action or practice in question; (2) identify the key *actors* in terms of the context-specific functions or capacities in which they are acting; (3) distinguish which *attributes* (or information types) are in play; and (4) ascertain *principles of transmission* governing information flows.

The heuristic provides a way to compare entrenched practices with those introduced by novel systems: Does the new system introduce different actors into the information flows? Does it offer access to new types of information? Does it shift the terms under which information flows, for example, from "with permission of data subject" to "with payment to service provider"? Detecting differences flags the need for further examination and evaluation. Although the default favors entrenched informational norms, which are presumed to support settled social values and interests, a thorough normative evaluation may favor the patterns that emerge when novel technical systems interject in an information flow.

Conducting a normative evaluation of novel flows involves three layers: one covers *interests*, a second, *general ethical and political values*, and a third, *context-specific ends and values*. The first two are subjects of a large and growing literature on privacy that probes harms and benefits of various systems, devices, and sociotechnical practices they occasion. Beyond interests, it considers whether values are threatened, for example, through unfair discrimination, threats to autonomy, chilling of speech and association, and so forth. Less evident, however, is attention to context-specific aims and values, such as health outcomes and fair allocation of benefits in a medical context, productivity in the workplace, and trust and safety within the home.

To start, context must be counted. Are we considering practices within clinical medical settings, health and fitness communities, places of work, or families? Background context will make a profound difference to how disruptive information flows are experienced by individual users and affect the significance and meaning of these patterns of flow. The perturbations of novel practices on an entrenched system may be positive indeed if they allow for a better realization of the relevant values. Such are the hopes pinned, in the United States and elsewhere, on a contemporary build-out of a health information infrastructure to improve healthcare delivery, medical outcomes, cost efficiency, and public health and well-being. But because health self-tracking is not limited to the healthcare context, a fact emphasized by developers and promoters, it is crucial to locate the various contexts of use in order to track and evaluate relevant information flows and positive and negative impacts on those respective contexts.

**Descriptive Evaluation**

In what follows, we draw on the Contextual Integrity heuristic to examine and evaluate privacy concerns in the development and use of health self-tracking in one context: that of the workplace. In our view, this case portends a worrisome trend deserving close attention and mitigation. Leading fitness tracking companies may cultivate new markets not only by selling their products and services directly to the public via retailers, but also by embedding them into existing health and wellness infrastructural ecosystems. For example, an employee might receive a free or discounted fitness tracker from her corporate employer as a benefit of enrolling in the company's workplace wellness program, or on the condition that it be worn for a particular event, such as a fitness competition, or to demonstrate mastery of a particular fitness goal, such as a daily step count average. Its use may even establish eligibility for discounted insurance premiums under the terms of a health-contingent wellness plan. Under a different model, employees might voluntarily use health self-tracking devices to log personal fitness metrics and share this information with colleagues by uploading it to company servers or otherwise making it available for viewing by fellow employees. One firm, for example, aims to track correlations among the fitness, productivity, and happiness of its employees by integrating health, project management, and social interaction data collected in-house and externally (Finley 2013). Are these flows disruptive? And if so, are they morally defensible?

**Context.** To begin, we place these practices in the overarching context of the workplace. Information flow patterns may vary from one workplace to the next (e.g., Mount Sinai Hospital, the CIA, or Walmart), and may be shaped by physical *layouts* (e.g., corporate offices, open warehouses, or delivery routes) and specific employment *junctures* (e.g., job interviews, performance assessments, or insurance pricing evaluations). However, there are salient common characteristics, including workplace hierarchies and purposes, which yield a significant set of expectations common to most.

**Actors.** For purposes of our analysis, data *subjects* are tracked company employees. *Recipients* of information generated by tracking systems may include the data subjects themselves, their peers, bosses, and other company officials, and persons associated with the tracking devices and affiliated service providers. Device and service providers also function as data *senders*, as might other entities acting as intermediaries for the purpose fulfilling a program's mandate, such as third-party wellness administrators or insurers who analyze and aggregate user data and send it back to their corporate clients.

**Attributes.** The type of information in question could vary from case to case, depending on the devices and systems used, as well as the programs and policies of particular workplaces. It might include daily step count or other activity metrics, weight and body mass index (BMI), foods eaten, calories consumed, heart rate, sleep quality, asthma symptoms, mood, and more. This information may be linked with other identifying information, such as demographic data or company department, or with workplace productivity metrics. In general, self-tracking systems provide an unprecedented degree of detail about health information.

**Transmission principles.** When evaluating new patterns of flow brought about by novel technology-enabled practices, the focus is on alterations to these terms from baseline to novel practices. Because these may be highly variable from case to case, findings will likewise vary. Further, since health self-tracking may introduce new types of information, there may be no baseline practices with which to compare. Taking Fitbit as an example, a subject's activity data are automatically uploaded to the Fitbit server as a condition of using the tool. This principle is different from one governing a subject's self-reporting of mood, energy levels, or alcohol consumption, or of one governing a subject's uploading of data from another self-tracking tool, such as a connected weight scale, glucose monitor, or food tracker. Here, differences hinge on whether data sharing is mandatory or optional, automatic or manual, and also whether it is subject to regular renewal and cross-platform integration.

The character of transmission principles is also determined by employers' general policies, including the terms of employee insurance plans, remuneration programs, and oversight practices concerning health-related lifestyle habits. A leap to automatic transmission of a continuous stream of biometric data for assessment against fitness requirements, for example, would be a huge departure from more settled practices, such as optional, scheduled, in-person biometric screenings with an employer's insurance provider representative. Variation may also be introduced as a function of specific agreements between employers and third-party tracking companies, or between employers and employees. Employers might impose contractual obligations on service providers to make employee information available for analysis. Or, companies might impose "softer" obligations to their employees, communicated as ideals of corporate good citizenship. One company official remarked that health data collected by her company is "not used for anything at this time" and "we don't base any team decisions around it." However, she also noted that if a potential employee is turned off by lifestyle information sharing, "he or she may not be a good cultural fit for the company in the first place" (Nield 2014). This position does not appear to allow for a real choice as to whether to authorize transmission of information. Transmission principles would also govern an employer's policies on sharing employee data with parties outside the company.

**Normative Evaluation**

Privacy concerns that emerge in the wake of new technologies are often dismissed on grounds that "nothing has really changed" aside from better access, more efficient monitoring, or greater convenience. Such claims may comport with privacy understood in terms of the dichotomy of *private* vs. *public*, or subject *control* of information, or concrete *harms* suffered. The finer lens of Contextual Integrity, however, reveals a different picture. It flags alterations in information flows to which more reductive accounts are blind; it offers a rigorous account of these instead of vague charges of "creepiness," or, worse, of irrationality. In our two cases, but also generally for health self-tracking systems, Contextual Integrity reveals that flows are altered in all three parameter fields—actors, information types, and principles of transmission. Disruptions in any of these parameters, as noted earlier, may be vectors of privacy violation if they fail to meet the criteria of a normative analysis.

Of greatest significance is the new inclusion of employers as recipients of information produced by health self-tracking, which, in our view, inappropriately extends the reach of employers into the lives of employees. (We cannot ignore the irony of retaining the prefix "self" for these flow patterns, as well as those in which systems providers automatically interject their servers as repositories for tracked data.) Unlike prior employment history or performance outcomes, which may even be automatically tracked, health and lifestyle information penetrates into zones formerly reserved for family, friends, or physicians.

One could argue that employers are already expanding their role beyond merely writing a paycheck for work and supervising, managing, and mentoring workers (Henderson 2009). Employers no longer behave as mere *employers*, but additionally assume expansive roles of insurers, benefits providers, behavioral police, and cheerleaders for health, productivity, and happiness. Since employers are paying for health benefits and profit from healthful employees, they have an interest in encouraging healthy lifestyles and attention to fitness and other health metrics. But total involvement by employers may not equally serve employees' interests: continuous tracking may be experienced as illegitimate intrusion into personal life, generating worry and anxiety and preventing relaxation and rest outside working hours. Power differentials between employers and employees may be exacerbated, particularly if policies regarding onward distribution of data are unclear, raising questions about who will get access, under what terms, and with what results.

Researchers and social commentators have challenged incursion such as these into employees' lives. Legal scholar Katherine Stone, for example, calls them collapsed contexts, or "boundaryless workspaces" (Stone 2002), and warns of threats to workplace fairness, equity, and justice. Another legal scholar, Michael Selmi notes, "One of the problems we have in defining the proper space for workplace privacy is that it is no longer clear what work is about, what the boundaries of work are, or even what it means to be an employee. ... It is one thing to give an employer broad dominion over its own workplace but quite another to extend that dominion wherever the employee goes" (Selmi 2006).

Ways in which novel flows affect respective interests constitutes the first layer of analysis prescribed by Contextual Integrity. Presumably, employers' interests are served by producing a harder working, more resilient, and less costly workforce. Yet, for employees, this trend changes the "psychological contract" with the employer, jeopardizing the sanctity of spaces for relaxation, reflection, and experimentation (Stone 2002). It also expands zones in which employers may exercise power over their employees.

Especially worrisome is the prospect of workplace discrimination if an employer infers that an employee has (or may develop) an impairment that limits her ability to work, or increases health-care costs. In a recent study of contextual expectations of health information flows, Fitbit users strongly resisted employer access to health and wellness data (Patterson forthcoming). One research participant objected, for example: "I don't want an employer or a potential employer to go and find all my diabetes, all my blood pressure, blood glucose, and weight, and all this other medical information, and then say 'This guy's going to drive our healthcare [costs] up.' And so, I don't even get the interview because [a potential employer] has just tremendous insight into my health before he even contacts me." Further, research participants were keenly aware of associated harms, such as disadvantages in hiring or promotion processes. For example, they flagged that information about weight or eating habits may signal an inability to exert the kind of discipline and self-control that is valued in the workplace; that information about sleep cycles may signal poor productivity; that information about moods may signal depression or general instability or unreliability; and that information about family histories of diseases like cancer, diabetes, or heart disease may signal increased insurance costs and place them at risk of dismissal.

These fears are not irrational. In the early 1990s, Indiana's Best Lock Corporation, whose policy prohibited the use of alcohol, drugs, and tobacco both at and away from work, attempted to fire an employee for disclosing that he had once consumed alcohol at a bar with friends (*Best Lock Corp. v. Review Bd. 1991*). In 2007, Scotts Miracle Grow successfully dismissed a newly hired lawn-care technician for violating the company's nicotine-abstinence policy (*Rodrigues v. The Scotts Company, LLC et al. 2009*). And in the past few years, Methodist Hospital System, Baylor Health Care System, and Citizens Medical Center have announced policies against hiring applicants who use nicotine or whose body mass indices (BMIs) indicate that they are obese (Roberts 2014).

When considering impacts on ethical and political values, as directed by Contextual Integrity's second layer of analysis, questions of fairness are raised by employers evaluating workers on the basis of health, fitness, and lifestyle choices instead of exclusively on the quality of their work. A traditional understanding of the scope of workplace performance evaluation may encompass, for example, an assessment of an employee's skills, work output, productivity, efficiency, intelligence, originality, creativity, speed, reliability, consistency, honesty, meticulousness, and ability to work well with others. The introduction of health criteria into this space extends the image of the idealized "good" employee to someone who is fit, trim, and even-tempered, who sleeps well, and has few or no vices outside of work. Much as Henry Ford instructed dozens of investigators in his Social Welfare Department to spontaneously visit the homes of employees and flag behaviors that violated company policies, such as gambling, drinking, taking on lodgers, and engaging in sexual relations outside of marriage (Maltby 2008), today's employers implement strict policies related to their actual and future employees' offsite behaviors (Roberts 2014).

Heightened scrutiny and uncertainty may lead to what James Hoopes calls "management by stress" (Hoopes 2005) and what University of Kansas Professor Jerome E. Dobson refers to, with respect to GPS tracking of employees, as "geoslavery" (Dobson and Fisher 2003). Professor Jeffrey Rosen cites sociologist Erving Goffman for the proposition that job tensions are increased when employees must perform under constant scrutiny (Rosen 2001), and notes that workers "experience a dignitary injury when they are treated like the inhabitants of the Panopticon" (Rosen 2001). These outcomes do not merely spell harm, but threaten values to which the majority of Americans subscribe, such as individual autonomy, respect for persons, just deserts, and fair treatment.

Even if workplace wellness programs are framed as voluntary, employees may experience economic pressure to participate, social pressure to conform, and diminishing privacy expectations. Law professor Scott Peppet notes that when disclosure of personal information is economically attractive to employers, as well as inexpensive, easy, and common, pressure builds to disclose. Those who resist may be seen as withholding negative information from the community, and thus be stigmatized and penalized (Peppet 2011). Consequences of nonparticipation in health-tracking programs can be serious: by charging unequal health insurance rates to differently situated individuals unless they achieve a particular set of health outcomes, wellness programs place an extra burden on the poor, the sick, and those genetically predisposed to obesity, heart disease, diabetes, and alcoholism. Consequently, those in greatest need are likely to be worst served by such developments.

The third layer of Contextual Integrity analysis looks for impacts on ends and values of the workplace context. One consideration is organizational stability, achieved through the cultivation of a well-trained, secure, and established workforce; trust in the fair allocation of rewards, reflecting workplace effort, education, training, ability, and interest; and structural arrangements that support workplace cooperation. Social psychologist Roderick Kramer, for example, observes that small gestures, such as the elimination of storeroom locks or time clocks, or the presence of policies encouraging employees to borrow company equipment on the honor system, may signal to employees that they are trusted by their managers, and in turn facilitate an expectation of reciprocal cooperation, "creating a shared common knowledge of the ability of the players to reach cooperative outcomes" (Kramer 2006).

Individuals are adept at "neutralizing" undesirable surveillance by avoiding situations in which they will be monitored, by masking or distorting their identities, and by plainly refusing to participate in data collection activities (Kramer 2006). Gary T. Marx notes that workers whose productivity is evaluated, for example, by the number of typed keystrokes they produce in a fixed period of time may resort to distorting their true efficiency by pressing a single key for several minutes at the end of the tracked window, perhaps obfuscating their output in order to preserve autonomy or to bring their scores into alignment with performance expectations (Marx 2003). The overseer of a state health policy center recounts that students forced to participate in annual fitness "weigh-ins" thwarted intrusive surveillance by wearing ankle weights under their jeans (Hoffman 2015). Defensive strategies such as these may undermine the social and economic success that the programs are designed to promote. Employees subjected to real-time health monitoring may similarly find ways to subvert surveillance in a cat-and-mouse struggle to achieve a discounted annual health insurance premium, and, in so doing, adopt an oppositional stance within the workplace.

These forecasts of dysfunctional work environments resulting from the insidious surveillance of health tracking data, while merely speculative, are drawn from insights into the outcomes of other forms of close worker surveillance. One final observation concerns not so much workplace as workforce. An efficient distribution of human resources would match individuals with work to which they are best suited. The United States prohibits various forms of workplace discrimination, such as discrimination based on gender and race, for primarily ethical reasons. But there is also an efficiency argument to consider. Prejudicial hiring means that the most qualified candidates will not necessarily be chosen. Similarly, short-term prejudice against well-qualified candidates based on health factors might threaten the overall quality of the workforce. Although we are not in a position to validate this point with economic data, Contextual Integrity would suggest examining this thesis as an aspect of the third layer of analysis concerned with contextual goals and values.

## Mechanisms for Protecting Privacy

We have focused primarily on norms of flow supported by a context-based analyses of disruptions posed by health self-tracking systems. In this section the question is practical: what means do we have for enforcing, shaping, or merely encouraging the adoption of practices that comply with these norms? We fear that individuals have unrealistic expectations of the legal system's ability to protect privacy in health-tracking data. They may incorrectly believe self-generated information to be medical in nature, and therefore covered by health privacy laws. Let us take a hard look at existing offerings, and consider gaps and vulnerabilities as well as hopeful future directions for closing these gaps.

### Architecture

Any design plan must consider what information is collected, how it is collected, how it is used, to whom it flows under which circumstances, how it is to be stored and maintained, and under what circumstances it is to be destroyed. Design choices, therefore, reveal a privacy and security footprint for any system (Lessig 2006). By the same logic, a consideration of these choices allows the creators of a system to design for privacy and security. Health self-tracking systems may incorporate several junctures at which data are collected, processed, and disseminated. For example, under one model, after information is collected automatically from fitness bands, it is transferred to a company's cloud server where it is integrated with information from other devices and services. Data are algorithmically analyzed according to various health metrics and then is delivered to personalized dashboards on the service provider's website, or on the user's smartphone app. These data can then be pushed to the end-user's friends via social media feeds, pulled by software developers and their customers via application programming interfaces (APIs), and shared with affiliated third-parties or other business partners, such as employers or insurance companies. Designs that seem inevitable to non-expert users are rife with choices that could have been made differently: for example, whether gathered information first pauses on a user's system so that she may decide whether to allow or restrict onward flow, and whether she may then engage with permissions that are built into a system in order to customize access to others at her discretion. We mention information collection and transfer points to highlight that each juncture presents an opportunity to apply privacy-enhancing design choices. If we want architecture to embody these constraints, we must first know what the constraints are, and we should have the means of holding designers accountable for their design choices.

### Law

Much of United States privacy law has developed in relation to concerns about specific technological advances that surprised and worried the public. When Samuel Warren and Louis Brandeis wrote their now-famous 1890 *Harvard Law Review* article advocating for the legal codification of a "right to be let alone," they were reacting to a particular confluence of new inventions and business models that concomitantly enabled new information flows: flash photography, printed newspapers, and other machines allowed for the easy collection and rapid circulation of visual images—and accompanying crops of unseemly gossip—that threatened to make real the ominous fear that "what is whispered in the closet shall be proclaimed from the house-tops" (Warren and Brandeis 1890).

Beginning in 1903, a number of privacy laws responsive to the indignities that Warren and Brandeis foreshadow emerged from the courts and legislatures. However, unlike its European counterparts, the United States Congress has repeatedly declined to pass omnibus federal privacy legislation. Rather, it has enacted a suite of sectoral laws applying to information circulating within particular contexts such as education, health care, and finance. Additionally, administrative agencies such as the Federal Trade Commission (FTC) and the National Telecommunications Information Association (NTIA) codify and enforce regulations on relatively cabined aspects of social life, such as consumer protections or telecommunications.

Although often criticized as insufficiently protective of privacy, the United States' sectoral regime implicitly acknowledges that privacy hinges on contextual factors, imagined and valued by persons in somewhat different ways, at different times, against more powerful norms-governed backdrops. Indeed, individuals often organize their social behaviors to avoid violating norms underlying these contexts. Thus, even for identical data—say, one's weight or blood pressure or heart rate—selective sharing and withholding of information is not only acceptable, it is often socially obligatory. Health confidences made to one's family, friends, or physician, for example, would be odd and perhaps unwelcome if made to one's employer, first date, or PTA board, and could result in discrimination, rejection, or ostracism.

As a general matter, regulation of health self-tracking is problematic because much of the information collected and processed by commercial sensors and app companies is closely aligned with, and sometimes identical to, data collected in the traditional medical context, but its privacy and security are not specifically subject to privacy regulations relating to health care. One might imagine, for example, that privacy rules associated with the Health Insurance Portability and Accountability Act (HIPAA) would be a promising avenue for protecting privacy in relation to health self-tracking data. However, health self-tracking information does not usually fall under the purview of HIPAA because the law is limited to discrete health-care relationships, rather than health information. Where physicians or insurance plans are subject to restrictions regarding storage and distribution of their patients' or customers' health self-tracking data, commercial actors and others who hold the same data are not. In the cases of health information in the employment context or in home life, protections afforded by HIPAA do not necessarily apply.

Employees do enjoy some limited protection through a patchwork of legal rules designed to mitigate employment discrimination and coercion. For example, in the case of workplace wellness programs that qualify as HIPAA-covered health plans, HIPAA's privacy provisions allow employers access to only "summary health information" without employees' written consent. Under HIPAA's anti-discrimination provisions, employers are required to limit the size of the financial incentive they offer to employees for participating in wellness programs, and to offer a reasonable alternative to employees who do not qualify for a program. The consent provision in these instances is laudable, but in practice it weakens HIPAA restrictions. Under one insurance company's employee wellness program, for example, an Authorization and Purchase Form for the Fitbit pedometer asks employees to sign a waiver consenting to their step counts being viewed by their human resources department, and to avow honesty in earning step counts and performing walking activities (United Healthcare 2012). Further, outside the rubric of bona fide wellness plans, the voluntary disclosures to companies, such as those undertaken in the spirit of workplace camaraderie discussed earlier, are not covered by HIPAA.

The Americans with Disabilities Act (ADA) and the Genetic Information Nondiscrimination Act (GINA) offer protections against workplace health-based discrimination, but these are also only partial. The former limits circumstances under which employees may be required to submit to medical examinations or meet a health standard in a health-contingent plan; the latter prohibits discrimination based on genetic information by group insurance plans and by employers. However, ADA provisions are only triggered if a disability is in play. Commentators generally believe that the ADA offers little recourse against discrimination based on lifestyle factors (Roberts 2014). Employee information protected by GINA is limited to genetic information and does not include information about sex, age, race, or ethnicity that is not acquired via a genetic test.

Focusing on federal law covering the employment context, we find that employees currently have few rights against private sector employers who engage in various forms of monitoring or tracking. Private sector employers are permitted to search and engage in widespread surveillance of employees, including testing for drug use, tracking employees' phone calls and texts, monitoring employees' whereabouts via GPS or RFID tags implanted in clothing or badges, and subjecting applicants or employees to honesty and personality tests. A number of states have "lifestyle statutes" that protect the rights of employees to engage in lawful activities outside of the workplace during nonworking hours, such as smoking and drinking alcohol. These statutes, however, are not absolute and allow employers to take action if the behavior in question conflicts directly with essential business-related interests, or violates a legal or contractual agreement with the employee. The common law privacy torts may offer some protections to employees but are similarly limited in scope. The tort of Intrusion Upon Seclusion, for example, provides a cause of action where one's solitude or seclusion is intentionally intruded upon in one's private affairs or concerns in a manner that is "highly offensive to a reasonable person" (American Law Institute 1977). With rare exception, narrow interpretations of "private affairs or concern" provides an employee with little recourse to monitoring that can plausibly be related to employment, even if undertaken outside of the workplace, and any careful "reasonable person" analysis must take into account changing social practices ushered in by new technologies.

### Policy

As we have seen, existing legal protection covers only thin slices of the domain of health-tracking systems. Outside the scope of these legal regimes, the practices we discuss fall within the regulatory framework of commercial actors whose business involves collecting and using personal information. In the United States, this extensive landscape ranges over companies that collect information in the process of providing other goods and services to those whose business *is* information. Under the dominant regime, self-regulation, companies declare self-fashioned information practices through privacy policies and, in principle, are held accountable to these by government agencies, primarily the FTC.

Regulatory bodies and advocacy organizations have urged companies to base their voluntary policies on the Fair Information Practice Principles (FIPPs), a set of principles first articulated in the 1970s by a Committee of the U.S. Department of Health, Education, and Welfare and, virtually simultaneously, adopted by the Organization for Economic Co-operation and Development (OECD) (Regan 1995). Developed in response to deep worries over the growing use of computerized database technologies, the FIPPs have been a cornerstone of government and commercial privacy regimes, and have been formulated to provide clear notice to individuals regarding the collection, use, dissemination, and maintenance of data, to articulate the purpose or purposes for which this information is collected and used, to retain only data relevant and necessary to accomplish those purposes, and to seek consent for these practices or departures from them. Further, data quality and security provisions should ensure that stored information is accurate, relevant, timely, and complete, as well as protected from loss, unauthorized access or use, or disclosures through appropriate security.

Companies wishing to present themselves as conscientious actors generally adopt the rhetorical stance of presenting privacy policies clearly and implying that individuals are free to consent to them, or not. The reality, as critics have pointed out, is a far cry from the ideal. Even when policies are written with care and with fidelity to FIP principles, they are notoriously long and difficult to understand. Ample research shows that most people do not read privacy policies and that when they do, they do not grasp them. Often, policies are deliberately written broadly enough to encompass a vast range of behaviors—present and future—in order to protect companies against legal liability through inadvertent violations.

A major source of weakness is that the FIPPs offer primarily procedural and not substantive protections. The FIPPs are envisioned to level the playing field between more and less powerful actors by codifying procedural rules of fairness and by providing a measure of control to individuals through consent mechanisms. In practice, however, companies may be virtually unrestricted in the practices they follow, so long as they declare them in those same policies that no one reads or understands. This opens a great loophole, important to mention here, but discussed in greater detail elsewhere (Nissenbaum 2015). An alternative regime for regulation suggested by Contextual Integrity is through substantive rules derived from ideal contextual informational norms.

Regulators are aware of self-regulatory shortcomings and have recently contemplated how best to approach the protection of consumer data, including self-generated health information. In May 2014, for example, the FTC held a seminar examining the collection, use, and distribution of health data generated by consumers and corporations outside of the traditional health-care context (Federal Trade Commission 2014). And the White House's 2015 Consumer Privacy Bill of Rights discussion draft is prescient in recognizing that consumers often engage with technology differently as a function of the social contours of a particular business sector or environment (White House 2015). However, respecting context requires an awareness of what consumers expect from a particular social context, and of what is at stake when information flows are disrupted (Nissenbaum 2015).

## Future Work

As health data move into employment and other spaces, previously unheeded relationships will need to be regulated by a suite of complementary legal, policy, and architectural formations. Whether externally imposed or voluntarily adopted, new privacy-protective measures will benefit from a clear articulation of the nexus between data flows and contextual values. Contextual Integrity provides a procedural roadmap, but data are needed to inform fuller analyses that can translate to concrete and appropriately nuanced architectural, policy, and legal solutions.

Fundamentally, a commitment to contextual privacy demands a commitment to radical transparency. The onus here is on companies to self-disclose, and on legislatures to require self-disclosure. Transparency is vital because it is impossible to critically evaluate a new program without fully understanding what consumer information is collected and how it is used. Thus, "radical transparency" in our view entails explicit point-to-point flows of information that reveal precisely what type of information is disseminated, to which parties, and under what conditions. Technologists, social scientists, philosophers, policy analysts, and legislators each have a role to play in defining and shaping the contours of these developing systems. Particularly needed are careful audits of information collections and flows, coupled with social science research that delves deeply into users' expectations for (and practices with) new technologies. When combined with a clear identification and articulation of contextually grounded values, this resulting knowledge base should enable the identification of gaps between actual and desired legal protections, and from there, the enactment of laws regarding which informational transactions should proceed, and under what conditions.

To illustrate: in the situation of health self-tracking data making its way into the employment context, the patchwork of legal regulations on employers are so sparse—and employees so thinly protected—that new federal privacy regulations of actors distributing and receiving data may be warranted. This could take many forms, including developing a broad federal statute protecting employee privacy rights with respect to surveillance, of which health surveillance is but one type; extending HIPAA to cover employers, per se, regardless of the administrative path (e.g., wellness plans tied to insurance plans) through which health information is collected; or even by removing health information from the workplace entirely. Defining the character of these types of safeguards requires a much closer look at all facets of the information flows we have identified in this chapter, bolstered with a careful analysis of how these restrictions operate in practice.

One reasonable approach may be to segregate identifiable data that users provide for a given purpose, such that it is available for use in that context but unavailable for migration to other spheres. For example, early empirical work suggests that individual and familial genetic profiles, mental health characteristics, sexual and reproductive health histories, and lists of current medication would be strong candidates for mandatory segregation in the employment realm, hedging against invasive health surveillance practices that threaten the mutual respect between worker and employer that underlies a cooperative workplace. In practice, this would place most health information flows to employers off limits by default, and perhaps render them inalienable even with employee consent.

But it may be the case that users sanction certain types of information flows if conditions are met, such as nearly absolute assurances of data de-identification and encryption, or a strongly restricted recipient list, or a demonstrably and solely prosocial use of the data. For example, some individuals may choose to permit the distribution of data for research purposes when it is closely tied to the topic of the research study (e.g., genomic data for gene sequencing research). It should not be assumed that in doing so they are giving either explicit or tacit permission to use the data for generalized research purposes. Similarly, individuals may tolerate or even embrace certain data flows to medical personnel such as physicians, but only under the conditions that the information be held in the strictest of confidence and be distributed only when it may reasonably help another medical professional assess a condition that the data subject wants evaluated.

What conditions underlie trust in health information flows in an employment context? To fully grasp these issues, certain information must be acquired, such as how employees who are subject to such scrutiny respond to it in practice, for better and for worse. What are employee fears? What would an ideal information-flow system look like to workers in different types of employment situations? Under what conditions, if any, would employees and colleagues be privy to which types of health data, and why? But before these questions can be answered, we are sorely lacking fundamental factual details:

- What, in practice, are the myriad channels through which health data are currently introduced into the workplace, and how, precisely, do different types of tracking technologies alter the nature or number of these channels?
- What is the exact nature of the data that get introduced through each channel? What, if any, of this information is combined with additional data to reveal new insights about employees? If this occurs, what additional data are accessed and analyzed, and what insights are revealed?
- How and by whom are various categories of information stored, analyzed, and shared within a variety of workplaces? With what personnel? And which informal, and thus potentially unexpected, information dissemination routes are active in various types of workplaces—for

instance, observation, small talk, and gossip—and what are the ramifications of these for employees?

Without these facts, information-sharing practices are subject to ongoing speculation, as is a full accounting of their positive and disruptive effects.

Note that in laying out the need for future empirical work, we are not suggesting that either wholesale resistance to or adoption of new self-tracking technologies is the correct course of action—but rather, that solutions will benefit more from specific knowledge than from broad sketches. We encourage entities that conceive, design, and deploy domestic health self-tracking systems to consider relevant cultural and social contexts in order to more effectively incorporate notions of contextually appropriate information flow into privacy-protective legal and policy frameworks.

## Summary

In this chapter we have argued that novel information flows brought about by new health self-tracking practices are best evaluated according to the ends, purposes, and values of the contexts in which they are embedded. Health self-tracking practices may, for example, heighten power disparities between data subjects and recipients that undermine the internal stability of spheres such as employment, where autonomy and freedom from surveillance are necessary to create a productive and harmonious workforce. In others not discussed here, such as the domestic sphere, they may introduce new and unexpected secondary surveillance by third parties, potentially unsettling caregivers in a sensitive environment where trust and security are paramount. Self-tracking tools and practices thus provide intriguing opportunities to explore the philosophical roots of information flow conflicts that occur in relation to specific actors at particular times in a variety of places: within our bodies, our workplaces, our homes, and more.

As society collectively adjusts to value evolutions brought about by new technologies, the proper roles of technologies, laws, and policies may also shift. Architectural, legal, and policy solutions governing the entities collecting and distributing information should be considered in light of, and developed to complement, regulations of entities receiving it. One site of contestation may warrant broad changes in federal regulatory oversight; another may be more effectively addressed through the adoption of new technological or policy practices that maximize information flow transparency and thus better enable individuals to operationalize and enrich values in a particular sphere. Empirical work is essential to the creation of solutions that serve the needs of individuals and society and better enable underlying social norms to weather rapid technological advancements into the future.

## Note

1. The authors contributed equally to this work and are listed in alphabetical order.

## References

American Law Institute. 1977. 652B Intrusion Upon Seclusion. Restatement of the Law, Second, Torts.

*Best Lock Corp. v. Review Bd.*, 572 N.E.2d 520 (Ind. Ct. App. 1991).

Dobson, Jerome E., and Peter F. Fisher. 2003. "Geoslavery." *IEEE Technology and Society Magazine* (Spring): 47–52.

Federal Trade Commission. 2014. "Spring Privacy Series: Consumer Generated and Controlled Health Data." https://www.ftc.gov/news-events/events-calendar/2014/05/spring-privacy-series-consumer-generated-controlled-health-data. Accessed August 10, 2015.

Finley, Klint. 2013. "What if Your Boss Tracked Your Sleep, Diet, and Exercise?" *Wired UK*, April 18. http://www.wired.co.uk/news/archive/2013-04/18/quantified-work-citizen. Accessed August 10, 2015.

Henderson, M. Todd. 2009. "The Nanny Corporation." *University of Chicago Law Review* 76: 1517–1611.

Hoffman, Jan. 2015. "'Body' Report Cards Aren't Influencing Arkansas Teenagers." *New York Times*, August 10. http://well.blogs.nytimes.com/2015/08/10/body-report-cards-arent-influencing-arkansas-teenagers/?_r=0. Accessed August 10, 2015.

Hoopes, James. 2005. "The Dehumanized Employee" *CIO Magazine* http://www.cio.com.au/article/165305/dehumanized_employee/. Accessed August 8, 2015.

Kramer, Roderick. 2006. "Social Capital in the Workplace." In *Social Psychology of the Workplace*, ed. Shane R. Thye and Edward J. Lawler, 1–30. Oxford, UK: Elsevier JAI Press.

Lessig, Lawrence. 2006. *Code v2*. New York: Basic Books.

Maltby, Lewis. 2008. "Whose Life Is It Anyway?: Employer Control of Off-Duty Smoking and Individual Autonomy." *William Mitchell Law Review* 34 (4): 1639–1649.

Marx, Gary T. 2003. "A Tack in the Shoe: Neutralizing and Resisting the New Surveillance." *Journal of Social Issues* 59 (2): 369–390.

Nield, David. 2014. "In Corporate Wellness Programs, Wearables Take a Step Forward." *Fortune,* September 3. http://fortune.com/2014/04/15/in-corporate -wellness-programs-wearables-take-a-step-forward//. Accessed August 10, 2015.

Nissenbaum, Helen. 2009. *Privacy in Context: Technology, Policy, and the Integrity of Social Life.* Palo Alto, CA: Stanford University Press.

Nissenbaum, Helen. 2015. "Respect for Context: Fulfilling the Promise of the White House Report." In *Visions of Privacy in the Modern Age,* ed. Marc Rotenberg, Jeramie Scott, and Julia Horwitz, 152–164. New York, NY: The New Press.

Patterson, Heather. Forthcoming. "Contextual Expectations of Privacy in Self-Generated Health Data." Working Paper. New York University.

Peppet, Scott. 2011. "Unraveling Privacy: The Personal Prospectus and the Threat of a Full Disclosure." *Northwestern University Law Review* 105 (3–4): 1153–1203.

Regan, Priscilla M. 1995. *Legislating Privacy: Technology, Social Values, and Public Policy.* Chapel Hill, NC: The University of North Carolina Press.

Roberts, Jessica L. 2014. "Healthism and the Law of Employment Discrimination." *Iowa Law Review* 99:573–635.

*Rodrigues v. The Scotts Company, LLC et al.* (639 F. Supp. 2d 131 2009).

Rosen, Jeffrey. 2001. *The Unwanted Gaze: The Destruction of Privacy in America.* New York, NY: Random House.

Selmi, Michael. 2006. "Privacy for the Working Class: Public Work and Private Lives." *Louisiana Law Review* 66 (4): 1046–1056.

Stone, Katherine V. W. 2002. "Employee Representation in the Boundaryless Workplace." *Chicago-Kent Law Review* 77 (2): 773–819.

United Healthcare. 2012. "Healthy Directions 2012 Employee Fitness and Wellness Program, fitbit [sic]." http://www.airbornemx.com/benefits/HEALTH%20AND%20WELLNESS%20AMES%20PROGRAM%20detailed%20communications%20to%20employee%20-%20HRA,%20fitbit,%20and%20health%20rewards.doc. Accessed October 25, 2014.

Warren, Louis D., and Samuel D. Brandeis. 1890. "The Right to Privacy." *Harvard Law Review* 4 (5): 193–220.

White House. 2015. "Administration Discussion Draft: Consumer Privacy Bill of Rights Act of 2015." https://www.whitehouse.gov/sites/default/files/omb/legislative/letters/cpbr-act-of-2015-discussion-draft.pdf. Accessed February 28, 2015.

# 6

# Disruption and the Political Economy of Biosensor Data

Brittany Fiore-Gartland and Gina Neff

Science and Technology Studies has long held that the frames and definitions designers give to new tools matter enormously for how users initially receive and ultimately modify those tools. Discourses are powerful forces in technology design, shaping, for instance, how gender and racial inequalities get designed into technologies (Suchman 2002). The startups working in biosensing and self-tracking present a case to examine the role that power plays in the discursive process of framing new technologies. One frame often used for defining new data tools and services includes their abilities for "disruption," or the perceived ability of technologies to upend the status quo of power within established industries and social institutions. In this chapter we present findings from our research in the startup environment in the relatively less-regulated consumer wellness field and the more closely regulated field of mobile medical applications. We use two cases of health data innovation to present possibilities for scholars and practitioners to think about both the processes and discourses of disruption, and how these discourses might affect the design and use of new technologies. Our goal here is not to make normative or evaluative judgments about the roles that disruption discourses play in society. We hope to show that disruption discourses limit how people imagine technologies could bridge existing social contexts and categories. Disruption limits such vision by overlooking the distinct roles for and relationships around data across contexts. People can have different expectations for data within and across different social institutions (Fiore-Gartland and Neff 2015). Social institutions, too, produce the tools and methods for making data intelligible across different contexts. However, the framework of disruption at best ignores social institutions and at worst maligns them. These ways of talking about disruption help to reproduce existing institutional power, even as people use the term disruption to describe how they purport to change, replace, or disrupt those same power arrangements.

This chapter examines how two popularly held expectations for disruption—democratizing power and democratizing access—function to replace one set of existing ideas about power with another. We argue that the disruption label masks the underlying friction and fuzziness of contested visions for social institutions. The discursive work of the label "disruptive innovation" marshals support for the technology development process. These disruption discourses matter because they can cut off possibilities for some markets, while attempting to remake the existing world in an image that dismisses a new set of power relations. Disruption as a discourse is a form of negotiating power—a form that often privileges one mode (for example, of access to data or markets or expertise) over another. In their most extreme form, disruption discourses use the concepts of democracy and democratization as ways to describe technological change, and in doing so ascribe social power to technological change in a teleological, deterministic way: if we say a technology disrupts power by bringing democratic access to data or power, then the technology will be democratic.

We focus here on the disruption discourses in health-care innovation in general and biosensing in particular, which both use contradictory notions of the process of social change that new technologies initiate. Disruption discourses suggest that hardware and software can or should stand in or substitute for social power. These disruption discourses present an imagined process in which all the details managed by government, policies, and citizens—the social actors in existing institutional power—would be fully accounted for, and still wholly dismissed or wholly encompassed by the disruptive change. In this way, disruption functions as an ideology that imagines that new technology can displace institutional power, and yet forecasts a new world that relies on new social arrangements for power, arrangements that do not exist or are not yet specified. The disruption discourse embodies a friction between different notions of democratization, which has implications for how technology is designed in relation to institutions. Disruption discourses shape how technologies are encoded with values about existing laws, regulations, norms, and social practices.

We examine two startups confronting the U.S. Food and Drug Administration (FDA), 23andMe, makers of a direct-to-consumer genetics test, and Biosense, makers of a mobile urinalyses app, uChek. First, we look at the common disruption discourses around new kinds of biosensor data.

Then we examine how the FDA ruled against these two companies that used disruption labels to market biosensing technologies and services. While neither case is settled at the time of this writing, we argue that thinking through how disruption is used shows the multiple and conflicting roles data play within social institutions and the social process that intermediates those roles. We argue that these multiple, conflicting roles are important for making data understood across different social settings. They trouble a simplistic disruption ideology and suggest a complexity in how data are framed, used, and regulated by norms, expectations, laws, and social arrangements. Finally, we suggest what our research implies for technology designers, health innovation advocates, and scholars, and what it contributes to the critiques of disruption that are emerging.

## Disruption as a Discourse

Disruption is used to explain the trajectory of what has occurred and predict what will happen in the future. The concept has roots in Clayton Christensen's much-popularized theory of disruptive innovation (Christensen 1997, Christensen and Raynor 2003). Christensen argues that new market entrants disrupt incumbents by creating a new market with cheaper and worse products that fill a need that other companies had ignored or overlooked. Disruptive innovation describes a process by which a new product or service that is worse than the status quo along some valued dimensions eventually displaces the industry incumbents. The incumbents are displaced because they ignore other sets of values. Nor do they understand how to expand their market. The idea is that industry incumbents are so busy focusing on their "sustaining technology" and meeting the needs of their mainstream customer base that they do not see the disruptive innovation coming (Christensen 1997). Christensen and Raynor (2003) distinguish between "low-end disruption" and "new market disruption," describing how disruptive innovation can take root either within the bottom of the market for customers that don't want or need the full performance valued by other customers, or within entirely new markets that are not serviced by incumbents. A disruptive innovation in an established field does not so much improve on incumbents' products as it offers simplicity, affordability, and accessibility.

Disruption has evolved into an ideology of the technology industry. Conferences such as TechCrunch Disrupt present a model of change defined around a clear choice: "Disrupt or be disrupted." Within the ideology of disruption, new technology is thought to generate a whole new plane of competition for market incumbents. The disruptive innovation label is widely applied to many new technologies, causing even Christensen to express skepticism to its ubiquity (Bennett 2014).

Critics point out that while disruption may function as a theory of why businesses fail, it does not help explain why and how industries change (Lepore 2014). Critics of Christensen and the ubiquitous use of the disruption label suggest that disruption may not apply outside of technology and manufacturing. Christensen himself advocated for disruption to describe what he sees as necessary changes for health care and education. However, large government actors who wield regulatory power are among the incumbents. Mehta (in this volume) provides an example of how disruption can be used to understand the trajectory of Apple's QuickTake digital camera—a significantly more affordable and lower-quality new product—in which Apple positioned itself as a disruptive innovator because camera industry incumbents ignored new markets. Mehta argues that the health-care industry, distinct from the camera industry, doesn't just ignore the newcomers to the market; they try to regulate and stake their claim to emerging markets, even when they aren't actually providing services in those markets. Disruption discourses rely on the assumption of free markets, but in actuality, civic and public stakeholders and social factors shape how all businesses and industries work. However, disruption discourses suggest futures that are at least partly outside of social institutions such as governments and industries, even as these discourses are strongly invested with idea of changing those same social institutions from the outside.

Take as an example the prediction that health care's "outmoded institutions" will be "replaced, soon enough, with new institutions whose business models are appropriate to the new technologies and markets" (Christensen, Bohmer, and Kenagy 2000). Here, health-care institutions are framed as singular coherent systems instead of syncretic, plural, and hybrid entities that we know them to be as demonstrated by a wide range of scholarship. While Christensen presents disruption as predictive, we would argue that this logic of disruption is less a prediction about what will happen with the introduction of new sets of technologies and data, than an attempt to define the space of innovation and the terms and timelines of institutional change. In other words, we argue that when people use the word "disruption," they seek to proscribe how society should adapt to innovation rather than predict how it will change. It is not a far stretch in that case to see how disruption discourses then shape the priorities of technology design and innovation in terms recognizable with the disruption ideology. The thrust of the remainder of our chapter examines how disruption literally changes the terms of debate for health innovation in ways that frame social problems and market failures as having possible technological solutions only outside of social institutions.

## Innovation and Disruption in Health Care

Our field research was at the intersection of health care and technology, two industries in the throes of infatuation with disruption discourses. Health care is often noted as one of the last industries to be disrupted by the digital revolution (Vaitheeswaran 2010). Disruption advocates argue that the U.S. health-care system is an incumbent industry that can be simultaneously displaced and transformed through market-driven and technology-enabled innovation. "Will Disruptive Innovations Cure Health Care?" This provocatively titled article coauthored by Christensen argues "disruptive innovations, small and large, could end the crisis—but only if the entrenched powers get out of the way and let market forces play out. If the natural process of disruption is allowed to proceed, we'll be able to build a new system that's characterized by lower costs, higher quality, and greater convenience than could ever be achieved under the old system" (Christensen, Bohmer, and Kenagy 2000). Here Christensen and coauthors frame the U.S. health-care system as inefficient and ineffective, fundamentally broken, unsustainable, and "the most entrenched, change-averse industry in the U.S." (Christensen, Bohmer, and Kenagy 2000). They suggest that disrupting health-care institutions will make health care both cheaper and *better* (ibid.). This, of course, is in contrast to a path of cheaper and worse that Christensen's model of disruption predicts for other industries.

One way people predict disruption happens in health care is through direct access to cheaper, consumer-grade technologies and data. The model of social change presented in technology demonstrations, advertisements, and founders' talks presented technologies as capable of transforming how doctors in clinics and hospitals provide care and expanding where care is provided. Communities of entrepreneurs, designers of data and technologies, and users within the startup environment of consumer health and wellness claim that a wide range of digital health technologies could enable pervasive, ubiquitous sensing of our bodies, our minds, and our behaviors, driving a revolution in how people know and care for themselves. These data-intensive technologies developed outside of conventional health-care institutions and follow a market-driven, consumer-oriented logic. Many are wrapped in "disruptive innovation" as part of their marketing. At the conferences we attended such as TEDMed, Stanford's Medicine X, and Health 2.0, people referred to Christensen's language of health-care disruption and Topol's (2012) "creative destruction of medicine." People there argued that consumer sensing and data technologies will undercut the status quo with affordability and accessibility; create new ecosystems for clinical care, personal health, and wellness; and democratize consumers' access to data and diagnoses. Disruption was thus described as a desirable goal, an end, even, of the work of technology implementation.

Yet in these presentations and discussions no one mentioned that disruption says disruptors provide current customers with a worse product compared to that of incumbents. Entrepreneurs presented disrupting health care as a goal, but rarely did they include details on what new kinds of power or what new middlemen would emerge from the ruins of disrupted industries. Nor did they include timelines for how disrupted socio-technological arrangements would reconfigure. The majority of these so-called "disruptive innovations" are not focused on the work of negotiating changes to social power—key, we would argue, to any institutional transformation. Nor do they account for how institutions learn, adapt, and evolve. In the disruption ideology, it is a quick and complete process, not one with intermediate steps, involving players and stakeholders from within and outside of social institutions.

Christensen's disruption framework sees newcomers as those who "sneak in from below" to displace incumbents (Christensen, Bohmer, and Kenagy 2000). Health-care disruption, however, is often talked about as contradictory institutional processes. By this we mean improving or streamlining the services of incumbents' (hospitals, clinics, regulators) *while simultaneously* displacing or making redundant those services such as diagnoses, expertise, or clinical visits. This begs the question of who exactly is the incumbent to be disrupted and whether disruption best characterizes the changes that innovators are working toward.

These tensions around the definitions of disruption and ends of innovation are evident at the line between health and wellness data. The number of health technology companies and the number of health and fitness apps and devices are booming. Big data and personal analytics are increasingly popular venture capital investments. Rock Health, a digital health accelerator, reported that in 2014 digital health funding exceeded $4 billion, and for the first time the digital health industry surpassed total medical device venture funding (Rock Health 2015). However, there are few effective ways to aggregate, integrate, and use the abundance of personal data being collected and little work to date on creating models to help bring that data into health-care settings. While data are seen as disruptive, there have been relatively few examples of how data-driven business models apply to health-care service provision.

Most of the health technology startup community envisions disruptive innovation emerging through the convergence of what might be termed classically medical instruments for diagnosis and therapy on one side and consumer-oriented information and communication technologies on the other. Disruption discourses position doctors, clinics, and hospitals as inefficient and sometimes unnecessary intermediaries between patients and their data. Analogous to how Day and Lury (chapter 3, this volume) describe discourses around data as reassembling of the fiction we tell ourselves about the dividing line between the individual and the social, the disruption discourse reinscribes distinctions between social institutions and individuals. Another part of the disruption discourse is that a host of disruptive innovations enable self-monitoring and self-diagnostics, liberating health care from the confines of the clinic, while recreating, in effect, a data ecology of information, expertise, and analysis. Health and wellness management in this technological imagination becomes an *always-on* activity that exists everywhere the consumer is (Price Waterhouse Cooper 2012), blurring spaces of health and wellness in everyday life.

Our point is not to judge whether disruption is a reliable way to predict the effects of innovation in health care, but rather to critique the important discursive work disruption does for health-care technology design. What is at stake is a socio-technical negotiation process that represents and reproduces technologies along with the scripts and contexts for their appropriate use. This matters for two reasons. First, these configurations and scripts continually reshape boundaries between categories of medical and nonmedical, health and wellness, patient and consumer, and device and data. Second, these shifting distinctions have important implications for how health functions in practice within existing social institutions. How this is accomplished discursively is what we turn to in the next section.

## Disruption as the Democratization of Power and Access

For health care, disruption is said to bring about the democratization of power and access: individuals' access to information and tools empowers them to act for themselves, challenge expert knowledge, and shift power relations between doctors and patients (Eysenbach 2008; Hardey 2001; Topol 2012). In disruption discourses *democratization* is used in different ways with different implications for existing social institutions. Democratization of power refers to the empowering of laypeople through their data and technology to shift the power of medical expertise and entrenched actors in the health-care system. Democratization of access refers to the increased access to health care by putting medical information, data, and technology in the hands of laypeople, not health-care workers, often with the goal of providing care to underserved populations through decentralized means.

There is an idealization of data's democratic potential, though, that puts patients and consumers "at the center of action-taking in relation to health and healthcare" (Swan 2012a, 97). "Patient engagement" and "patient empowerment" are often tied to the process of providing new digital technologies and data to directly to individuals (Barello, Graffigna, and Vegni 2012; Eysenbach 2008; Swan 2012a). Such an empowered patient is the result of the shifting of trust and power away from social institutions and toward individuals and consumers. This idea of the empowered patient relies on the full participation and activation of consumers to drive these changes (Topol 2012). Empowerment, then, emerges first from individuals having access to personal and personalized data and second from individuals being able to act on their data. This discourse refers to users as sources of data and innovators around their own care solutions. For example, "e-patient" Dave Brokhart organized a movement calling to "give me my DAM data" to push health-care organizations to make their records open to patients, removing barriers to individuals' access to their information.

In the consumer narrative of democratization in health, individuals' access to information and tools of digital production empowers them to act in the service of their own health and wellness and to challenge and evaluate expert knowledge. In the process this access is predicted to disrupt the status quo configurations of institutional power (Eysenbach 2008; Hardey 2001; Topol 2012). Henwood et al. (2003) point to the dominant discourse of "rights" inherent in the emergence of consumer health informatics and to the emergence of Gidden's "reflexive consumer." The concept of "reflexive consumer" bears the assumption that individuals want to take more responsibility for their own health beyond the standard visit to the doctor. As the authors point out, this is not the case with all individuals: "'Rights,'" they note, "carry 'responsibilities'" (604), and from this perspective empowerment serves to shift a burden of responsibility away from institutions onto individuals (see, for example Rose 1999).

Disruption advocates see digital health tools and data as empowering consumers by reducing or removing mediation that is perceived as necessary or wasteful, and thereby enabling the consumer to perform activities such as diagnosis, monitoring, experimentation, and data sharing outside of clinical and scientific settings. This is sometimes described as do-it-yourself or "DIY medicine," where consumers can autonomously conduct an array of at-home diagnostic testing and Internet-based medical information searching (Khosla 2012; Swan 2012b). We call this process *disintermediation*, and democratization in disruption theory relies on disintermediation. In other words, for disruption to be democratizing, direct access to personal health data must empower individuals to change their behavior, make informed decisions about their health care, and actively engage particular research or drug development agendas. It does this, however, by taking out the middle.

Scholars point to the corollary neoliberal logic of responsibilization, in which the "power" to act is also construed as the responsibility to act (Henwood et al. 2003; Lupton 1997; Mol 2008). In the realm of digital health, the democratization of technology and data and the empowerment of the user are promoted as two sides of the same coin. Around this theme of democratizing power emerge very different configurations of the so-called "empowered" user and scripts for that use in relation to institutional power. This leads to very different configurations of the user in relationship to empowerment and to different configurations of how empowerment is defined in each context. Thus, disruption discourses attempt to redraw professional and occupational boundaries, relationships, and previously held notions of expertise, responsibility, and authority. Many consider consumer attitudes and technologies to be essential for disruption in health care because they will bring (free) market logic to entrenched hierarchies and generate a participatory culture. For example, Sue Desmond-Hellmann, CEO of the Bill and Melinda Gates Foundation and former chancellor of the University of California–San Francisco (UCSF), describes how the democratization of information shifts power from the institutions of medicines toward patients and consumer: "If the hierarchy of doctors are the only ones that have that power, that puts patients at a disadvantage. The power dynamic as a partner, as someone who has a stake in it, is different. Think of how much power you have every time you go to a consumer store" (Desmond-Hellmann 2013). Hellmann's reframing of the patient as a "consumer" with choice and buying power is an essential part of how this disruption discourse manifests a particular narrative of democratization. This frame configures users as empowered within a market-driven logic of choice (Mol 2008). Yet this consumer logic of choice means the patient bears a greater responsibility for managing his data and then navigating the implications of that data. Users, here, are autonomous and naturally inclined to be responsible for optimizing their own health, self-managing their care, and producing, sharing, and creating value with their personal health data. In disruption, the work of institutions is outsourced to individuals.

For entrepreneurs and technology designers, the discourse around "disruptive innovation" and "creative destruction" has generated a vision of consumer-oriented products, configuring the user as a consumer rather than a patient and health-care professionals are often completely left out of the equation. This vision may fit squarely within calls for disruptive innovation, but it is shaped by the perception that designing for consumers is much easier and less regulated than designing for the health-care system, which requires much more investment up front to comply with FDA and other institutional interoperability standards.

A new product does not need to seek approval from the FDA if it does not make any explicit promises or claims about diagnosis or treatment. For example, an app to help diabetics track data on their blood glucose levels would not need FDA approval as long as the company provides sensing with approved medical devices and keeps data distinct from any medical advice, diagnosis, or interpretation. This regulatory environment creates a disincentive for technology designers who might have otherwise built applications to inform both physicians and patients. Instead we see the disruption label applied to the explosive growth in consumer-targeted applications aiming to provide personal data separate and distinct from the "incumbent" health-care system.

Disintermediation is a process that assumes that medical expertise can be codified in other forms to disrupt institutions. Algorithms, thus, are framed as cheaper, more accessible, simpler, and only slightly less skilled doctors of the future (see, for example, Khosla 2012). Disruption discourses fundamentally overlook the work required for data to move across contexts. This is what doctors do when they interpret general lab results for particular patients within their own particular medical treatment protocols. They translate data from one realm (the lab) to another (the patient's particular case). A wide array of different practices is needed to make data sensible, meaningful, and actionable. Our two cases that follow illustrate this.

## Disruptive Data: 23andMe and uChek

The trajectory of the personal genetics testing company, 23andMe, embodies the frictions between the notions of democratization of access and democratization of power. On November 22, 2013, the U.S. FDA issued a warning letter to 23andMe demanding the company halt the marketing of its direct-to-consumer (DTC) genetic test kits until the service received FDA device marketing authorization. In response, 23andMe stopped providing any "interpretation" of health risks with the test results they provided to their customer, and solely provided "ancestry-related information and raw genetic data" while trying to win FDA approval (Fiore-Silfvast 2014).

Until the FDA letter, 23andMe provided a service that straddled a deliberately blurred line between health care and personal wellness, between patient and consumer, and between device and data. Similar to a host of other consumer mobile health applications and biosensors (i.e., Fitbit, Basis, InsideTracker, uChek), personal genetic testing is situated at the edge of regulation, pushing the boundaries of unregulated consumer health and wellness products by offering a model of consumer experience with health data that takes place outside of conversations with health-care providers and outside of health-care institutions, leaving the consumer to make sense of and manage the implications of data in everyday life (see Kragh-Furbo, Mackenzie, Mort, and Roberts, chapter 1 in this volume). As a data service, 23andMe occupies a gray area between offering consumers entertaining, educational, nonclinical interpretations of their DNA and offering personalized health-risk information that could have medical implications and be clinically actionable. For instance, 23andMe's marketing campaign before the FDA censure included a TV commercial presenting what people learn from their 23andMe test results. One man says, "So that's why the sun makes me sneeze," right before another woman says, "I might have an increased risk of heart disease" (23andMe 2013).

The juxtaposition of these two statements demonstrates the challenge of regulation, which is not about the data per se; rather, it is about the expectations for what people will do and try to say with data. Advocates of 23andMe discuss clashes with regulators as evidence of the disruptive nature of their service. As 23andMe charts new spaces of personal health data intermediation in the consumer realm that make health predictions, the health-care industry and the regulatory bodies are framed as impeding progress.

The 23andMe case challenges the institutional frameworks for medical knowledge generation, which require clinical and analytical validation, while it also celebrates democratization of power enabled through a data ecology that constructs personal health knowledge and expertise as wholly outside of clinical settings. In addition to these mostly nonclinical uses provided through the test, there are increasing amounts of personalized information about health risks and drug responses that have medical implications that the FDA is then responsible for regulating. Individuals cite their right to know about their own genetic health risks and to participate in the ongoing process of discovery that operates ahead of clinical translation. But in doing so they bypass the traditional intermediation, or translation, of data by doctors and care providers. Genetic testing data become more "democratized," in the sense that consumers have disintermediated access to their own personal genetic information. Yet, without institutional support and integration into the health-care system, these data in the hands of consumers fall short of empowering consumers in the clinical realm.

Here we see the friction between democratization of access and democratization of power emerge. Access to information is not the same as the power to act upon it. On the one hand, disruption in the 23andMe case refers to democratized access to personal genetic testing and data and suggests that new relationships will emerge through which these data may flow. On the other hand, within existing regulations, data have implications for medical decision making. The time scale for these expected transformations is not discussed, which reinforces a discontinuous break and avoids discussion of the new work and structures that would need to develop. The case of 23andMe shows that the power to create medical knowledge and make medical decisions and diagnoses has yet to shift outside of the health-care system. While any new, emergent ecology would ostensibly replace existing institutional norms and hierarchies, what it looks like is kept deliberately vague.

Does 23andMe simply want to disrupt access to personal genetic testing or does its leaders want to disrupt medical expertise and institutional power in their role of providing medical advice? 23andMe founders framed their service as "potentially" relevant for health with medical implications. They are outside the current institutional norms, while still at the frontier of genetic scientific discovery. They represent their company as the future of health care because they provide personal genetic data. Without some interpretation, translation, or mediation, genetic data is meaningless to most people. In other words, the 23andMe version of disruption replaces one type of data mediation done by doctors and by clinics with a mediation role that the company creates for itself.

For the FDA, the target of regulation is the service of interpretation that 23andMe provides to consumers that links genetic data to health risks and drug responses, which may have clinical implications, rather than the data itself. The FDA's letter to 23andMe points to the marketing language the company uses to describe its services—including "health reports on 254 diseases and conditions"; categories such as "carrier status," "health risks," and "drug response"; and specifically as a "first step in prevention" that enables users to "take steps toward mitigating serious diseases" such as diabetes, coronary heart disease, and breast cancer"—as overreaching into clinical interpretation with medical implications. From a regulatory perspective, these intended uses for 23andMe data fall under the medical device classification, which presents an expectation that the algorithms and delivery system be analytically and clinically validated in particular ways and to particular levels of accuracy.

Even in a clinical context, however, 23andMe data are mostly not actionable. While the FDA claims that the test could lead to such things as "prophylactic surgery" and "chemo-prevention," this is not too likely as most physicians would conduct further clinical investigation, rather than act based just on 23andMe data. However, physicians will still be confronted with 23andMe data as well as a range of other patient data generated outside the clinic that they will have to decide whether to act on or not, with potential clinical consequences either way.

This contradicts the notion that disruption of health care is necessarily democratizing to both the access to information and the power to act. Those who produce and consume disintermediated health and wellness data will not only be figuring out problems for themselves, but also using these tools to confront institutionalized power within the health-care industry; asking for medical expertise and knowledge to help them make sense of "their" data; and seeking ways to recreate some of the familiar types of data mediation available within existing social institutions and the current health-care system. While they may use a label of disruption, 23andMe is offering something more complicated. By offering a version of disintermediated data to consumers they still benefit from the relationship of consumers and their care providers to make sense of that data and to act on that data. In other words, consumers are not "just" working out for themselves the implications of the data that they get outside of the health-care system. This is a key difference in how the FDA has viewed 23andMe's data and the company itself has framed the data. Disruption in this case is not about 23andMe offering a better service. Rather, the company is disintermediating something the health-care system cannot provide, delinking health data from medical interpretation. In the process, 23andMe's design of service worked to change social institutions by imagining that the genetic data 23andMe provides can be completely outside of a health system.

Taking a step back from this controversy, we see that the consumer health side of 23andMe's personal genome service is a relatively small part of the company's larger strategy, which is to amass enormous amounts of personal genetic data. Anne Wojcicki, cofounder of 23andMe, told *Fast Company* that they had a goal of enrolling twenty-five million people. When aggregated and linked with phenotypic data, such data could fuel unprecedented biomedical discovery and pharmaceutical development. The company's 23andWe research initiative invites consumers to participate in research because "23andMe isn't just about you" and "with enough data, 23andWe can produce revolutionary findings that will benefit us all." The FDA's regulatory focus in this initial controversy only scratches the surface of the range of regulatory and ethical questions around how to manage contested data valences across the multiple contexts for privacy and reuse of big data (see chapter 5, this volume). It grapples only with different interpretations of what genetic data points mean, by enforcing standards of verification, not yet with the multiple expectations for what data can do and how it will perform within different social contexts (see Fiore-Gartland and Neff, 2015).

23andMe's version of disruption places the company and the data it provides fully outside the existing social institutions of the health-care system. In contrast, there is already a market-driven and consumer-oriented culture around disintermediated health and wellness in urban India. There individuals engage in self-care and self-management using technology that performs as the intermediary. This is due to the fragmented private and public health-care systems often failing to meet the demands of consumers, growing health insurance penetration, and the increasing burden and awareness of chronic disease. Technological innovation in health care in urban India is often centered on creating more autonomy, control, and self-sufficiency for consumers within and outside the formal health-care system.

Consider the journey of a mobile urinalysis app developed by a startup in India that transforms the mobile phone into a lab. The mobile app with accessories uses urine test strips and a camera phone to analyze colors compared to a color-coded mat on which the strip is placed. The app claims to analyze more than ten different parameters including glucose, bilirubin, ketone, specific gravity, and pH. The use scenarios for this app are multiple. The first category of use is for at-home urinalysis for an urban Indian population increasingly burdened with self-managing chronic disease. The second category of use is in clinics and labs, too small to afford the gold standard auto analyzers, which serve Indian populations underserved by doctors, clinics, and hospitals.

Biosense released a downloadable iPhone app for uChek in the United States. The FDA issued its first-ever warning letter to a mobile app provider explaining that Biosense needed class II medical device approval for uChek. In essence, Biosense framed the data it provided as non-medical data, but regulators disagreed, seeking to regulate the medical interpretation of data. Scanaflo, a similar device, was designed in Silicon Valley with the intention of marketing to self-managing and self-diagnosing U.S. consumers, but unlike uChek, it underwent the FDA approval process. The difference between the two types of biosensing is relevant because it reveals the multiple visions for what the same technologies and data can be across different institutional contexts, motivated by different health-care problems and thus open to different kinds of regulatory interpretations.

## Disruption Discourses as Spaces for Development

Disruption may not function as a reliable prediction about what will happen in health care, but it does important discursive work, and thus shapes technology design. Disruption discourses shape the priorities of technology and data design, emphasizing potential consumers or markets rather than prioritizing health-care problems and social institutions of health care. Disruption discourses imagine data as capable of residing outside of social institutions and in the process fail to consider the mechanism that people look to for intermediation. Disruption discourses also imagine that access to data will enable people to act in particular ways, unrestrained by existing practices, norms, and laws.

The FDA has recognized the need for its policies to evolve in order to keep up with the pace of technological innovation and associated risk, developing a medical mobile application policy with a "balanced" approach that "supports continued innovation," while "assuring appropriate patient protections" (Foreman 2013). As of April 2014, of the tens of thousands of health-related apps on the market, the FDA had registered or cleared just over 100 as medical devices (MobiHealthNews 2014).

Disruption discourses in the U.S. consumer health context proscribe how medical and consumer data *should* travel between nonmedical and medical settings. In practice, however, data mobility was not supported by infrastructure to get consumer data into clinics or bring medical expertise to such data. The explosion of consumer-oriented biosensing has outpaced the development of institutions of sensemaking. Data do not move their own; rather, they require organizational structuring and intermediary labor to support the flow across stakeholder communities. Medical data produced in the consumer realm faced regulatory challenges as U.S. government bodies aimed to regulate medical devices, including medical interpretation or diagnosis, through FDA approval and regulated medical information. Without FDA approval what could occur in these new nonclinical sites and interactions was restricted, and the types of self-care available and the production of medical data via digital health technologies were narrowed, regardless of the promise or actuality of the innovation. Various forms of intermediation, such as care managers, nurses, and genetics counselors, would be needed to link home and clinic and to translate between medical expertise and individual cases. Disruption discourses worked in these cases to help imagine home and clinic as distinct and isolated spaces with respect to health data, not as places ready for the social and technological bridges that new kinds of data could have provided.

Thus innovations in these nonclinical spaces tend toward two paths. In order to count in both settings, companies can go the route of seeking approval from regulatory bodies in order to afford interoperability between clinical and nonclinical settings. Alternately, they can take the path of focusing on wellness and prevention-oriented measures and interventions that skirt medical jurisdiction by a hair. In the latter case, the metrics around fitness, diet, well-being, and interventions may provide data without complete medical interpretation or present disclaimers that the information is "not for medical advice." This shaky bridging of the divide between official medical information and self-help begins to challenge the boundaries of health and wellness. We have seen wellness metrics and interventions explode in this interstitial medical/nonmedical space, along with national policymaking that promotes health through prevention and through the medicalization of lifestyle and well-being outside of the clinic rather than through episodic clinical encounters and disease treatment.

These differently situated technological visions bring different configurations of users, appropriate use, and context of use that are important in shaping the processes of digital health innovation. Disruption discourses helped people to imagine the distinctions between categories of medical and nonmedical, health and wellness, patient and consumer, and device and data. And these distinctions had important implications for how tools were designed to collect data and data functioned in practice across communities.

At the intersection between home and clinic were social norms and regulations that were not clearly delineated, and 23andMe attempted to straddle, but not bridge, these institutional contexts for data. With a disruption discourse that promised more democratic data, 23andMe designed a data ecology outside of the current health-care system, but ultimately dependent upon it for sensemaking and actionability of the data 23andMe provides to its customers. Biosense imagined the context for direct-to-consumer health being as global as the market in Apple's iTunes App store, and the technology moving as easily.

Firmly planted in the direct-to-consumer realm, 23andMe's disruption discourse seeks to change the status quo in health care through providing access to a new class of data that defies previous definitions of health and wellness. In this way, 23andMe uses access to data to open a space where the company supplants the conventional oversight and curation of the medical establishment. 23andMe essentially makes a market for personal genetic data and places themselves at the center. Their disruption discourse frames this as democratization, tapping into patient rights and empowerment discourses. However 23andMe simultaneously represents the shift of power from medical institutions to a corporate body, not to individuals.

Biosense comes from a perspective on disruption that is oriented around creating affordable and accessible health care for all, in a place where these gaps are stark. These technologies are imagined as innovations emerging from the massive demand and particular constraints that characterize other health-care settings in the developing world, in this case, India. The disruption discourse of Biosense holds that affordability and accessibility comes through democratizing access, disrupting the market for more expensive and less accessible ways of obtaining urinalysis. In their India development context, there was not a clear, entrenched health-care incumbent, and thus not the same notion of the democratization of power. Yet as uChek came to the United States the company found it was up against institutional powers that meant uChek was then framed as disrupting. Digital health advocates celebrate technology innovation as individual empowerment; yet within the disruption discourses empowerment is a process of individualizing the labor of data, placing the responsibility of achieving the appropriate health and wellness in the hands of the consumer (literally). As one author phrased it, individuals become "the CEOs of their health" through their expanded capacity to interface with devices and software algorithms (Khosla 2014). There is enormous possibility for people to use data-driven health innovations for a soft form of resistance (Nafus and Sherman 2014). However, disruption discourses make it harder for these innovations to work with and within existing social institutions as opposed to against them. At this point in health-care innovation is *disruption* doing more harm than good?

## Implications for Scholars, Designers, and Biosensing

For many consumer health advocates what is at stake in this controversy is the FDA trying to curtail their individual rights to access their personal health data. Communities of patient rights activists and advocates for consumer-driven disruptions in health care are demanding the liberation of all different types of personal health data from the constraints of clinical and medical settings and the return of that data into the hands of consumers. Information such as physician notes and medical device data have been the target of advocacy campaigns to create more access for patients and consumers.

So-called disruptive, data-intensive technologies in personal health and wellness, including emerging consumer biosensors, rely on an assumption that more data in the hands of consumers will lead to better health and wellness and that these data-intensive practices represent the future of health care. This assumption tends to overlook questions about the longer-term costs and benefits of innovation. There are many examples where worse/cheaper is not necessarily better for patients or health care. The assumption also ignores the central role of power for making data across multiple social settings. It also diverts focus from developing the personal genetic testing within health-care systems—systems that are much more hybrid and plural, more entrenched, and yet more adaptive than the way people frame these systems within disruption discourse.

We have demonstrated how data move from consumers across contexts to suggest that disruption discourses shape how consumer uses of data are imagined in the context of other social institutions. The attempts at disruption in health care corners technical innovation into a narrowly scoped context, in which its uses are circumscribed within a both nonclinical and consumer-oriented health and wellness context. Disruption discourses in health and wellness have already inspired challenges to distinctions between categories of medical and nonmedical, health and wellness, patient and consumer, and device and data. In circumscribing a context and design space that is just a hair before medical or that conflates health and wellness, as many of these technologies do, companies aim to escape the institutional and organizational implications of their design, such as regulatory policy, liability, and organizational capacity building. For technology designers, disruption discourses may limit their ability to create solutions with existing social institutions in mind.

Common frames in technology design presume that technology is capable of standing in for a whole host of organizational structures and institutional power. These discourses discount the multiple intermediaries that data need and the work that is required for data to be meaningful in different settings. In other words, when technology designers talk about data as disruptive they emphasize consumers, and often narrowly scope design around individual users, not multiple social contexts. This popular user-centered design approach in consumer health and wellness ignores the intermediation of data or where data resides and the organizational and institutional contexts for data. As biosensing becomes a consumer phenomena, how and where the data will go will continue to be an issue. When a technology is framed as disruptive, then the questions concerning where the data will go, who will evaluate it, and how it will help people work within the social institutions that exist are left unanswered.

Disruption discourses do powerful work in the design of data systems by imagining two things that are impossible to do simultaneously: cutting out a middleman while integrating seamlessly all the parts of the middleman's very system that will soon be made obsolete. This is where the discourse of disruption falls apart. Disruption discourses ignore the fact that data require mediation, even as disruptive services and technologies rely on new kinds of integration and new data mediation to work. Disruption presumes convergence on which institutional arrangements and configurations of power are to be transformed, and the expectations about institutional arrangements are articulated in the form of expectations for data. However, rather than see disruption as a challenge to social institutions, perhaps social theorists should remember that data always require norms, practices, and routines for sensemaking, meaning, and action. Perhaps the time is right to put data as disruption aside in favor of data as a social institution.

## References

Barello, Serena, Guendalina Graffigna, and Elena Vegni. 2012. "Patient Engagement as an Emerging Challenge for Healthcare Services: Mapping the Literature." *Nursing Research and Practice*. doi:10.1155/2012/905934.

Bennett, Drake. 2014. "Clayton Christensen Responds to *New Yorker* Takedown of 'Disruptive Innovation.'" *Bloomberg BusinessWeek*. June 20. http://www.businessweek.com/articles/2014-06-20/clayton-christensen-responds-to-new-yorker-takedown-of-disruptive-innovation#p1. Accessed August 18, 2015.

Christensen, Clayton. 1997. *The Innovator's Dilemma: When New Technologies Cause Great Firms to Fail*. Boston: Harvard Business School Press.

Christensen, Clayton, Richard Bohmer, and John Kenagy. 2000. "Will Disruptive Innovations Cure Health Care?" *Harvard Business Review*. https://hbr.org/2000/09/will-disruptive-innovations-cure-health-care. Accessed August 18, 2105.

Christensen, Clayton, Jason Hwang, and Jerome Grossman. 2008. *The Innovator's Prescription: A Disruptive Solution for Health Care*. 1st ed. New York: McGraw-Hill.

Christensen, Clayton M., and Michael E. Raynor. 2003. *The Innovator's Solution: Using Good Theory to Solve the Dilemmas of Growth*. Boston: Harvard Business School Press.

Desmond-Hellmann, Sue. 2013. "Attention Stressed-out Docs: Can the Consumer Be the 'Cavalry' That Rescues You?" TEDMED Talk presented at the TEDMED, Washington, D.C., April. http://www.tedmed.com/talks/show?id=18047. Accessed August 18, 2105.

Eysenbach, Gunther. 2008. "Medicine 2.0: Social Networking, Collaboration, Participation, Apomediation, and Openness." *Journal of Medical Internet Research* 10 (3): e22. doi:10.2196/jmir.1030.

Fiore-Gartland, Brittany, and Gina Neff. 2015. "Communication, Mediation, and the Expectations of Data: Data Valences across Health and Wellness Communities." *International Journal of Communication* 9: 1466–1484.

Fiore-Silfvast, Brittany. 2014. "Ethnography in Communities of Big Data: Contested Expectations for Data in the 23andMe and FDA Controversy." *Ethnography Matters^*, February 17. http://ethnographymatters.net/blog/2014/02/17/ethnography-in-communities-of-big-data-contested-expectations-for-data-in-the-23andme-and-fda-controversy/. Accessed August 18, 2105.

Foreman, Christy L. 2013. "Health Information Technologies: Administration Perspectives on Innovation and Regulation." Statement before the Committee on Energy and Commerce, Washington, D.C. http://www.fda.gov/NewsEvents/Testimony/ucm344395.htm. Accessed August 18, 2105.

Hardey, Michael. 2001. "'E-Health': The Internet and the Transformation of Patients into Consumers and Producers of Health Knowledge." *Information Communication and Society* 4 (3): 388–405. doi:10.1080/713768551.

Henwood, Flis, Sally Wyatt, Angie Hart, and Julie Smith. 2003. "'Ignorance Is Bliss Sometimes': Constraints on the Emergence of the 'Informed Patient' in the Changing Landscapes of Health Information." *Sociology of Health & Illness* 25 (6): 589–607.

Khosla, Vinod. 2012. "Do We Need Doctors or Algorithms?" TechCrunch. January 10. http://techcrunch.com/2012/01/10/doctors-or-algorithms/. Accessed August 18, 2105.

Khosla, Vinod. 2014. "20-Percent Doctor Included: Speculations & Musings of a Technology Optimist." http://www.khoslaventures.com/20-percent-doctor-included-speculations-and-musings-of-a-technology-optimist. Accessed August 18, 2105.

Lepore, Jill. 2014. "The Disruption Machine." *The New Yorker*, June 23. http://www.newyorker.com/magazine/2014/06/23/the-disruption-machine. Accessed August 18, 2105.

Lupton, Deborah. 1997. "Consumerism, Reflexivity and the Medical Encounter." *Social Science & Medicine* 45 (3): 373–381. doi:10.1016/S0277-9536(96)00353-X.

MobiHealthNews. 2014. "103 FDA Regulated Mobile Medical Apps." http://mobihealthnews.com/research/103-fda-regulated-mobile-medical-apps/. Accessed August 18, 2105.

Mol, Annemarie. 2008. *The Logic of Care: Health and the Problem of Patient Choice*. New York: Routledge.

Nafus, Dawn and Jamie Sherman. 2014. "This One Does Not Go Up to Eleven: The Quantified Self Movement as an Alternative Big Data Practice." *International Journal of Communication* 8: 1784–1794. ijoc.org/index.php/ijoc/article/viewFile/2170/1157.

Price Waterhouse Cooper. 2012. "Emerging mHealth: Paths for Growth." Economist Intelligence Agency. https://www.pwc.com/gx/en/healthcare/mhealth/assets/pwc-emerging-mhealth-full.pdf. Accessed August 31, 2015.

Rock Health. 2015. "Digital Health Funding: A Year in Review 2014." Rock Report. http://rockhealth.com/resources/rock-reports/. Accessed August 18, 2105.

Rose, Nikolas. 1999. *Powers of Freedom: Reframing Political Thought*. Cambridge, UK: Cambridge University Press.

Suchman, Lucy. 2002. "Located Accountabilities in Technology Production." *Scandinavian Journal of Information Systems* 14 (2): 91–105.

Swan, Melanie. 2012a. "Health 2050: The Realization of Personalized Medicine through Crowdsourcing, the Quantified Self, and the Participatory Biocitizen." *Journal of Personalized Medicine* 2 (4): 93–118. doi:10.3390/jpm2030093.

Swan, Melanie. 2012b. "Sensor Mania! The Internet of Things, Wearable Computing, Objective Metrics, and the Quantified Self 2.0." *Journal of Sensor and Actuator Networks* 1 (3): 217–253. doi:10.3390/jsan1030217.

Topol, Eric J. 2012. *The Creative Destruction of Medicine: How the Digital Revolution Will Create Better Health Care*. New York: Basic Books.

23andMe. 2013. http://mediacenter.23andme.com/blog/2013/08/05/poh_ad_campaign/. Accessed August 18, 2015.

Vaitheeswaran, Vijay. 2010. "A Very Big HIT." *The Economist*, November 22. http://www.economist.com/node/17493417. Accessed August 18, 2015.

# 7 Deep Data: Notes on the *n of 1*

Dana Greenfield

## Introduction: Enter Intensive Surveillance Unit

During my first Quantified Self (QS) Global Conference in 2013, I felt as if I was transported out of San Francisco's Presidio Park, into an alternate universe. This was not just because people introduced themselves as aspiring cyborgs, wore computers on their faces, or used technology to mitigate an anxious relationship to technology. It was the real-time, continuous EKG, heart rate, blood pressure, glucose data streams displayed on personal devices, displayed in clothing and accessories—sometimes shared publicly via social media—that felt alien. At the time, I had been toggling between California, where I was exploring personal informatics, and an intensive care unit (ICU) in New York, where my mother lay in a coma. The spaces of QS and the ICU may have shared the same data streams, but they were worlds away. I am a medical student turned anthropologist turned patient. For me, the meaning of data and numbers reverberated between these contexts, picking up new, uncanny resonances.

Digital and mobile health (what many call "dHealth" or "mHealth") devices that measure biometrics attempt to liberate and domesticate the powerful monitoring tools of ICU. In my mother's ICU pod, we followed the continuous monitoring of her blood and intracranial pressures (ICPs), her vital signs, her oxygen saturations. Every move of each number seemed to hold the entire past, present and future at once. We survived each day between the numbers, reading them like tea leaves. The cacophonous machines and data overwhelm the sensorium and mark the ICU as a place of exception in the hospital, the place of intense surveillance (if not care). I expected and experienced this as familiar, alienating, and frightening all at once. Comparatively, the continuous streams of biometric data in the bright ballroom in the verdant Presidio that day in San Francisco seemed out of place, even absurd. The willing self-surveillance of the mobile and (seemingly) healthy digerati appeared as bizarro actors in an off-kilter world, where the tools of exception (ICU) became the norm.

The ICU had strange visiting hours—three slots of two hours, each day—that made each visit a new encounter with my mother. Park the car. Sign in at the front desk. Take the elevator up. Round the corner to the ICU waiting room, where there was often a new cluster of people—a fresh tragedy. Pick up the phone to ask permission to enter. Walk slowly yet impatiently to her room. Gaze straight at the screens. Are the ICPs down? What about her fever? The numbers became a centerpiece of our conversations: explaining them to the medically naïve or discussing plans with the nurses and doctors when the numbers got out of control. My phone buzzed regularly with requests for the numbers from her friends. As if to fill in around the gaps between the digital intervals, we also held her hand, spoke to her, read to her, read to each other, and recalled memories with visiting friends and family. But when the simmer of conversation fizzled, she remaining mute, our eyes drifted up, away from her wasting body, to the screen. The data felt like they was saying more than we were, and certainly more than she was. They were charged with hope or devastation, depending on the day.

The tendency to treat data and technological images that decenter the whole person is often depicted as an effect of biomedicine's techno-scientific imperative (Gordon 1988; Koenig 1988). I recognized how easy it was to become complicit in this rendering of my mother. Yet, I felt powerless to resist it. Between caring for someone who was not there and hoping she someday would be, the numbers oscillated between hope and elusive control to empty promise, mocking and pointless; from something to talk about to the only thing people could talk about.

At the end of her life, my mother was the ultimate quantified self, a true *n of 1*—the idea of continuous, total biometric surveillance *ad absurdum*. It was between ignite talks (rapid presentations given by trackers) and trips to the demo booths at the QS conference when I received her last piece of relevant data: pictures of her brain that showed an absence of mind. Amid the numbers beating in the screen, the truth is that the mother I knew was not really there. The deluge of her data was a mere simulacrum of self, a maddening mirage that held up the possibility of life. There was no self there, at least not one that could be lived. As I wandered past happy cyborgs, giving off invisible, blue-toothed data exhaust,[1] I wondered what sort of self they thought they were quantifying. I wondered how they could possibly be so delighted to subject their daily lives to a clinical gaze that I had so badly desired to overcome?

This chapter addresses the implications of self-quantification in its relation to clinical quantification. By self-quantification, I mean those practices of keeping track of aspects of one's life, activity, or body. Some track actively, using a pen and paper, others with a custom-made spreadsheet. Other devices such as digital scales or home blood-pressure cuffs connect actively tracked data to a cloud server. Wearable devices, such as the Fitbit or a BodyMedia armband, or even smartphone applications such as Moves, enable continuous, ambient data collection (e.g., step count or heart rate). The complex and entangled relationship between medical and QS modes of accounting[2] is not yet well understood. In this chapter, I explore these trends in conversation with more traditional biomedical modes of accounting and quantification. I will then turn to the *n of 1*, a central tenet and practice of Quantified Self. The *n of 1* is where QS begins. Borrowing from scientific discourse, where the *n* signifies the number of participants in an experimental study, the *n of 1* suggests that knowledge can be gained at the scale of the individual. The *n of 1* rejects the requirements of large numbers of subjects for statistical validity and expert credentials, forging a new epistemology of health and being where the single case or person collecting data over a lifetime displaces the population as locus for knowledge and intervention. The *n of 1* unites the diverse QS community and collective, including the mood and productivity trackers, the health and bio-hackers, and the life loggers and personal data artists. Diverse practices and goals all start with the idea that the *n of 1* can and (maybe) must be asserted as the starting point for self-understanding, -expression, or -improvement. Providing a common ground for practice, the *n of 1* does different things for different people. Exploring the heterogeneity of *n of 1*, we can begin to understand how self-quantification entails a complex relationship to biomedical representation—from one that mimics and extends the gaze to another that undermines. In other words, the *n of 1* asserts itself as having legitimate access to self-knowledge and self-care, presumably unmediated by claims to expertise. How might the *n of 1* reproduce, undermine, or relate to critiques of disciplining and displacing practices of biomedical technologies (Foucault 2004)? What are the convergences and departures between the fog of data produced around my mother in the ICU and the instruments that enliven QS?

In what follows, I address the implications of QS as forming what I call *paraclinical* practice to describe what happens when clinical tools are redefined through their domestication. I take the *n of 1* as an experimental system[3] where new possibilities for the meaning and experience of health and illness ramify in surprising ways. Next, I describe extant and overlapping practices of medical knowledge production, against which the *n of 1* both wittingly and unwittingly casts itself. Last, I consider the polyvocal nature of the *n of 1* and what we might learn from it, as a space to rethink care and the clinical.

My analysis is based on fieldwork that was not restricted to QS as a community. I spent time at health technology conferences, and with entrepreneurs, an mHealth startup, a clinical tracking practice, and I continue to observe a large-scale dHealth research project in its attempt to innovate participatory research. What connects these diverse spaces and initiatives is that they are assorted experiments in health and care. Here the stakes of a health-care crisis (rising costs, chronic disease) are affixed to the ongoing management of wellness through behavior change. Health and care are not fixed concepts or achievements—rather, they are contested. The people and projects I encountered are in part a *response* to crises in health care. They participate in aspirational projects for what health and care might look like. Accordingly, they are also utopian projects, where, for example, health behaviors can be changed, medical mysteries can be solved, and self-knowledge, -mindfulness, and -awareness can be achieved.

## Medicine Inside Out

> You can't stop it. You can complain all you want, but you can't stop people from trying to make decisions and from trying to engage. … So, I have an AliveCor[4] and I told [the doctors] that. I ask for every copy of every interrogation of my implantable device and put that stuff up online and I ask for the insights and points of view of others who are laymen, a lot of times, and we're all sharing this stuff and talking about it, even though we may not be qualified to speak about this stuff. We're collecting [data]. … It's like the Aikido effect—when you use the energy of your enemy. … The idea is that you can't stop progress. Digital health devices will continue to appear. Will continue to create and figure out health platforms. We're going to continue to take [medicine] apart and decentralize control.
>
> e-Patient Hugo Campos, on a recent trip to a cardiology conference (interview 2014)

Campos is famous in the e-Patient movement for his ongoing quest for direct access to the data from his implanted cardio-defibrillator (ICD), a device that shocks his heart when it gets into a dangerous rhythm. For now, he has to visit his physician for any of the data collected by his implant. In addition to taking medications to keep his heart from jumping gears, he has tried to collect as much data as he can, using spreadsheets, an AliveCor® phone case, and a sleep tracker to get a handle on general health as well as dietary or behavioral triggers that send him into atrial fibrillation, for example. His own experiments and data gathering have led him to give up his occasional scotch or wine with dinner and question his caffeine intake, for instance. Showing me some of these data on his phone—in spreadsheets and EKG graphs—he lamented that these simple consumer devices were mere workarounds: "I have the ultimate class 3 implant medical device with high-fidelity data that is of clinical quality in me. It's ridiculous that I can't tap it, that I have to rely on these stupid little things that I have to move to my arm! The device knows when I go to sleep. The device knows my heart rate at every moment." MedTronic has yielded little in his effort to secure the data. Campos wages smaller battles now: refusing to allow remote monitoring by his physicians if he cannot access the data, asserting his participation in all clinical encounters, sharing his message on social media and at conferences as a patient-advocate, and seeking out electrophysiologists whose views are in line with his values of engagement and transparency.

Campos's ongoing collection of data from quasi-clinical tools is just one example of paraclinical practice: the self-tracking of biometrics, behaviors, and symptoms, borrowing the tools or metrics of medicine, and working alongside and even in opposition to formal medical practice. Paraclinical processes reproduce the clinic and its optics with a difference, as a departure. The *para* use of clinical techniques (an EKG, here) opens an adjacent space for producing new engagements with self-care and access to medical knowledge and data. The paraclinical sets the ground for the *n of 1*, operationalizing everyday experiences as sites for exploration and experimentation.

The paraclinical[5] is slightly distinct from the concept of biomedicalization, which is an extension of medicine to other human affairs (Clarke et al. 2003). Self-tracking can be a grafting of medical tools for personal means. Clinical techniques—from direct-to-consumer laboratory tests or "recreational" genomics,[6] to domesticated[7] EKGs or heart rate monitors—open to varied possibilities, from supplementation to subversion of medical authority. Instead of seeing the use of digital health technologies as the biomedicalization of everyday life, understanding them as part of paraclinical practice we see how recreating, appropriating, or grafting[8] tools of the clinical space enables continuities and ruptures in epistemologies. More than the domestication of clinical technologies, the creation of spreadsheets or graphs overlaps clinical renderings of personal and bodily experience.[9] These traces (Rheinberger 1997) potentially extend the logic of the clinic (e.g., remote monitoring). However, they also make an opening—as personal data for personal use—for reframing clinical questions and goals. The paraclinical, then, does not indicate that the clinic has necessarily or merely taken over the home, invaded it with its techniques or logics of pathology and risk.

What difference does the *para* make? The paraclinical hails a different kind of subject. Similar to a medical injunction to compliance (Whitmarsh 2013; Dumit 2010), QS as a paraclinical activity invites the subject to turn inward, becoming both subject and object of her own data-driven inquiry. In this process, the tools of subjectivation (Foucault 1986) (e.g., blood pressure cuffs, blood assays) are extrapolated from the clinic and are used for purposes outside of it. By taking up its tools, but not its claims to expertise, this is medicine turned inside out. Part self-help community, part user and maker group, part data politics agitators (Boesel 2013a), QS creates a community where members can reformulate the epistemic cultures of medicine and care.

## Getting the Numbers

Gathering quantified information has long been part of good clinical practice. "Getting the numbers," as it is called on the wards, in a contemporary clinical setting is part of using what Michel Foucault famously called "the clinical gaze" (1973). The clinic, he argued, enabled medical modes of perception and assessment to isolate disease in the depths of an individual body, apart from the context of familial and social life. Initially, a new science of pathological anatomy provided the gaze with its perceptive depth, revealing disease below the surface. The need to probe deeper, to isolate the seat of pathology, has manifested in the further development of diagnostic tools and devices from the x-ray to the blood pressure cuff (Ostherr 2013; Saunders 2010; Dumit 2003). Monitoring and quantifying in the hospital extend this gaze. In the hands of self-quantifiers—some nonpatients—these tools borrow but also depart from biomedical modes of quantified care, to which I now turn.

Self-quantification usually entails personal monitoring of symptoms or biometrics in ways the recall continuous or serial monitoring in the hospital. However, it was not until the early twentieth century when clinical tools were used to monitor, rather than diagnose. This shift in the use of data began with the rise of the patient-centric chart and the laboratory (Howell 1995; Berg 2004). The chart centralized clinical communication in an increasingly complex hospital, encasing the patient as an individual, data-intensive subject as well as an object of standardized documentation and treatment (Timmermans and Berg 1997; Berg 2004). Embodying the patient through diagnostic results and systematic notes, the chart and its data manifested Foucault's deep structure in actual clinical practice (Howell 1995). The patient's record and the graphs that began to pepper it were early modes of health data as "epistemic things" (Rheinberger 1997), vehicles for making new medical knowledge. More than an epistemic tool, the organization of the patient data into Subjective and Objective categories served to disavow the patient's claim to authority. Michael Taussig (1980) famously argued that such splicing alienated a patient from their own experience of illness, rendering them under clinical control. The politics of epistemic things matter for those who self-quantify, whose self-collected data flout such divisions.

Like clinical quantification, self-quantification may be viewed as an extension of risk and surveillance-based medicine, biomedicalizing daily life (Clarke et al. 2003). Getting one's own numbers—managing a daily blood pressure or activity level—means experiencing and minding individualized notions of risk (Castel 1991; Beck 1992; Gifford 1986; Armstrong 1995), rendering ostensibly healthy people into patients-in-waiting (Greene 2008; Dumit 2012a, b; Sunder Rajan 2006). No longer a binary, disease becomes distributed in a prodromal way, throughout the life course. This experience of vigilant risk is reinforced by pharmaceutical treatment practices where shifting thresholds for treatment—"prescribing by numbers" (Greene 2008)—further cloud wellness with risk. Many QS tools mobilize a risk-y gaze, keeping an eye on the horizon for disease. This can be part of a biopolitics where the individual is enjoined in self-care and discipline (Rose 2007; Petersen and Lupton 1996). However, self-tracking might be better understood not as disciplinary practice, but as forms of modulation and control (Deleuze 1992). As an ongoing, unfolding project of monitoring, data becomes an epistemic thing (Rheinberger 1997), where through its accumulation and repetition, differences and deviations can be recognized and managed.

Finally, the *n of 1* casts itself against evidence-based medicine (EBM) as another aspect of contemporary biomedicine. Having formally emerged in the 1990s, EBM spawned from the desire to rein in costs, hospital standardization movements, and a deeper paradigm shift from practicing medicine as an art to a clinical science (Timmermans and Berg 2003; Berg 1995). The hierarchy of evidence in EBM prioritizes large, experimental studies, while individual and nonexperimental knowledge recedes to the background. Guidelines are then developed from meta-analyses to apply the evidence to patients and populations. For proponents of EBM, this "gold standard" steers medicine away from a woefully irrational tradition of following judgment and experience. For opponents, it represents "cook-book medicine," blind to the nuance of individual experience, placing cost or statistical abstraction over care.[10] The hierarchy of evidence is both an epistemic and political tool, dividing sound fact from quackery.

The gaze of EBM is almost diplopic, with one eye on the patient and the other on the evidence (Sinclair 2004). As EBM privileges population-based data, the gaze moves laterally, panoramically, and probabilistically. Precision and personalized medicine is a response to this history of standardization and science-driven practice. The *n of 1* draws on the desires for precision, nonstandard medicine to assert a different mode of knowledge production altogether—the subjectively gathered objective data. As I explore below, the *n of 1* disrupts these dominant modes of clinical perception and care. For some, it is a gaze with heightened acuity. For others it instantiates a transition from experimental to an exploratory, big-data driven paradigm of medical knowledge production (boyd and Crawford 2012; Hey, Tansley, and Tolle 2009).

The *n of 1* grafts onto this varied history of medical accounting and perception, drawing on, interfering and colluding with the clinical gaze, itself multiple (Mol 2002). Now, I turn to the paraclinical gaze and various *ns of 1* I find there.

## From *n of 1* to *n-of-a-billion-1s*

> The n-of-1/n-of-billions idea will be vital to the program of Wikimedicine. Massive pooling of the granular but "pixelated" data from individuals creates a positive feedback loop, such that the overabundant granular data becomes more valuable and defined—transforming the extensive data to real information and knowledge that can ultimately be used to improve the health of individuals. The enhancement of health in a large number of individuals is the precursor to an upgrade in population health. This is how to connect the dots from the science of individuality to improving health on a large scale—a bottom-up approach that could not have been previously contemplated.
>
> Eric Topol (2012, 231)

> Imagine that you've got a gravitational field. … It's flat and a planet will be a big dip, and it takes a lot of energy to get out of the gravity well. These sorts of stories, the calorie in/calorie out story, the 10,000 steps story—are these energy wells. Good places to start. But how hard is it to get out of it? Quantified Self is a rescue ladder. … to get out of the deep imposed frameworks that are being dug

out under them and enables them to go to the higher flatter spaces where you could adopt or craft something that doesn't detract from [your] goals or identity.

Anne Wright, QS Organizer

These different yet related views of the *n of 1* tell us that there is a lot more going on with the *n of 1* than biomedicalization (Clarke et al. 2003). For Topol and others, personal big data is a big promise to transforming medical science and public health, finally delivering on precision medicine. For others, QS is a practice that serves a different purpose: finding personal answers to personal questions. Here, self-tracking and experimentation is more like a process of reflection and revelation, rather than a dataset, a natural resource to be mined by others. In this section, I discuss some of the many valences of the *n of 1* in QS as a nexus for the many stakes of self-quantification—from the epistemology to the politics of medicine.

Taxonomy of the *n of 1* would belie the fact that these meanings draw on each other, but I offer it as an exercise in outlining where experiences and practices overlap in a network of partially shared meanings:

In Table 7.1 are some of the varied meanings and practices I found associated with the *n of 1*. We find self-care as public health surveillance alongside DIY health and open data politics. Or, self-experimentation might be scientific democratization (citizen science or participatory research) or the vehicle for personal, life-long optimization.[11] I will survey some nodes in this semantic network, addressing those with particular implications for the practice and optics of medicine.

**Table 7.1**
*n of 1* taxonomy

| kinds of *n of 1* | Some practices, movements that relate |
|---|---|
| *n of 1* as aspirational self | *Homo experimentus*, Mindfulness tracking, Self-help, Optimization |
| *n of 1* as new public health | Anatomo-politics, Neoliberal self-governance, Compliance, Consumer health |
| *n of 1* as counter conduct | DIY health, Alternative epistemology, Participatory medicine, Data liberation |
| *n of 1* as care | Precision medicine, Self- and family-centered care, Participatory medicine |
| *n of 1* as collecting | Self-awareness, Mindfulness |
| *n of 1* as portrait | Narrative medicine, Data as mirror, Data as communication tool |
| *n of 1* as new science | Big Data, *Homo experimentus*, Citizen Science |

Who and what is served by personal data is a healthy debate in the QS community. What is at stake is partly captured by the distinctions between "surveillance" and "sousveillance"[12] or "self-tracking" and "other-tracking."[13] These concern power, privacy, and control, but there is more, too. The *n of 1* is the starting point for thinking outside given frameworks, or what Anne describes as "gravity wells." Put it another way, when faced with a problem, the *n of 1* seeks out a different kind of knowledge—insight that may not exist in a textbook or a diagnostic manual. Or in the case of the late self-experimentalist and psychologist Seth Roberts, the self is a fertile source for research idea generation,[14] seeing outside of the silos of given research. Starting from personal experience, QS enables a science of a different quality, not just a higher-resolution version of biomedicine. As a social, technical, and epistemic forum, the shared space of QS generates a kind of friction[15] where practices of care and inquiry co-mingle and potentially produce something unexpected and new.

## *n of 1* as Precision Medicine

As a medical futurist, Eric Topol (quoted earlier) forecasts that scaling up the *n of 1*—plugging the big data of personal informatics into the even bigger data[16] effort of EBM—will catapult us into the age of truly personalized, precision medicine. This "high-definition human" as Topol calls him, recalls a digitized upgrade of Foucault's anatomo-politics, where the political desires and drivers for better population management are operationalized at the individual level, just finer grained. In comparison, Foucault's anatomo-politics appear low-fi and modest. For precision medicine, the *n of 1* is an untapped natural resource,[17] which, once aggregated and deciphered, will unlock optimal health. As a departure from genomic personalized medicine of latter decades, where the genome was an inner truth to be known and disclosed, precision medicine indicates the need for ongoing interrogation and optimization of continuous flows of hyper-particular individual information. Throughout the Quantified Self Global Conference, some called for the need to upgrade the "quantified *self*" to the "quantified *universe*." Those with concerns over privacy or those who use QS as a set of techniques for personal growth did not necessarily share this sentiment.[18]

What exactly is the *n of 1* in this version of precision medicine? What kind of individual is posited here? Asking for a far more granular view of individual health through personal informatics, precision medicine asks not what is generally true of a disease or an intervention, but what is particular and provisionally true in a given moment for a given intervention for a given person. Precision medicine entails a tailoring of diagnosis, treatment, and prognosis given the *ongoing* and *continual* collection of personal data, mined at the *n of 1*, but also given meaning in aggregate. Unlike the aggregating technologies of EBM or the clinic, QS precision medicine does a different kind of work. Here—the crowdsourcing of personal health data—when the *n of 1* scales, it does not merely become the large *n* of a highly powered randomized controlled trial. Rather, the "*n of billions*" heard at QS and health technology conferences alike, is more like what I call *n of a billion 1s*. The return to large numbers is a return with a difference. The new crowd of *n of a billion 1s* differs from the "study population." For one, it is potentially ever expanding, not delimited, encompassing individuals without subsuming them to a group or average type. The open-ended nature of crowdsourced health data reflects the nature of the knowledge and subject produced—open to continual revision, improvement, and optimization. Relatedly, a new epistemic paradigm is embodied by the *n of a billion 1s*, where big data rather than experimental design produces insights[19] from ongoing datasets, where truth is an emergent property of information (Hey, Tansley, and Tolle 2009).

A different kind of subject emerges from the *n of 1* as a "high-def human" and the *n of a billion 1s*, one perhaps related to Deleuze's *dividual* (1992). The pixelated *n of 1* is a subject ever divided into finer granularity, but also whose partial datasets can be joined with others, in network, dividuated in data. The individual is no longer cast against and molded alongside the mass; rather the *crowd* and the *n of 1* melt into each other. In other words, the crowd or open data set[20] anticipates an *n of 1* that is already pixelated, made of similar stuff of the crowd, "interoperable" data points to be seamlessly joined to the *n of billions/billion 1s*. The ease with which personal data enters the cloud, fashions the "public" (RWJF 2014) into an "operable" or "bioavailable" crowd of untapped value (Cohen 2004). Kaushik Sunder Rajan (2005) described genomic research participants as "subjects of speculation," where multiple speculative processes (capitalism, experimental science, and predictive medicine) secured future market values. The *n of 1* scaled to *n of billions/billion 1s* adds to this guarantee to surplus value, where not only is future risk of illness a guarantor of future value, but also where the moment for modulation—real time—transposes the future into the present, over and over.

Topol's particular formulation of a "pixelated" human is just one of the strong views of how the *n of 1* enters into medicine. In concert with EBM, his *n of billions* searches for clinical truth from the aggregate. But are they both referring to the same thing? I argue that EBMs target and unit is the population, while that of precision medicine is the crowd, an aggregate of a *billion 1s*. The individual is articulated differently here. In EBM, the individual is considered in *context* of the evidence, whereas, in precision medicine the individual *is* the context. Is the pixelated individual a more complete understanding of the human? It might be the next best resolution or just a partial view, again.

Grasping for a pixelated human, something not lost to the crowd, is another such attempt to remediate this aspect of the clinical gaze. In the following sections, I will explore how the practices of *n of 1* among those in the QS community relate to the optics and epistemic values of medicine as well as attempts to pixelate the human in the service of the crowd.

## *n of 1* as Counter Conduct

It's not about big data or small data, it's about our data.

Gary Wolf, Founder, Quantified Self

In the late 1960s and early 1970s, feminist activists gathered in homes and community centers to teach each other how to a wield a speculum and mirror to do their own vaginal exams and to share personal stories. The latter served as "consciousness raising," where people connected across their personal experiences. The former aimed to wrest control of women's health from the medical establishment by teaching self-care. The "self-help clinic" was also a space of epistemic innovation, where both women's stories and intimate protocols started with the self as a partly oppositional, partly medical way of knowing. In *Seizing the Means of Reproduction*, Michelle Murphy (2012) describes such practices as *counter conduct*. These women did not renounce the tools of the clinic; rather they reappropriated them and forged their own technomedicine. As epistemic pioneers, they crafted new modes of objectivity,[21] exposing the "affective economies of technoscience," or "how capacities to feel, to sense, and to be embodied are valued within political economies of technoscience" (72). Put simply, feminist self-help placed affect—sharing narratives, examining bodies in an emotionally saturated space—at the center of credible knowledge making.

Quantified Self (unwittingly) recalls feminist epistemology by grounding the self as the starting point for knowledge. Self-tracking also qualifies as counter conduct when paraclinical practices open a space for challenging hegemonic medicine. This *n of 1* also shares with feminists the reformulating of affective economies science, where narrative and subjectivity (often on display at "show and tell talks") are similarly centered as epistemic virtues. Unlike feminist self-help, the *n of 1* is not overtly political.[22] Nevertheless, I use counter conduct as a frame for understanding paraclinical practices, where the *n of 1* is a vehicle for reassembling the hierarchy of evidence. Neither big, nor small, Gary's "our" data gestures at this move, sidestepping questions of scale to grounding epistemic legitimacy in the self by engaging narrative, affect, and politics of ownership, access, and control.

The QS tagline promises "Self-Knowledge through Numbers." Not better medicine through numbers. Not better public health through numbers. Not lower health-care costs through numbers. Mostly, QS leaders attempt to defend the space—conferences, websites, and meet-ups—from a takeover by the growing app and wearable industry. The presentation formula—"What did you do? How did you do it? What did you learn?"—reflects this mission. Here, logging weight by pen and paper or food by spreadsheet are techniques of self-tracking as much as a wearable biosensor. Tracking accommodates many goals, from passive, long-term data collection to active logging for mindfulness and behavior change. Centering the self serves more than personal needs. Self-experimentation can reframe epistemic values and politics, reintroducing affective attachments to scientific inquiry and seizing the means of (knowledge) production.

## "N=1, Loved by All"

In August 2014, friends of Seth Roberts—experimental psychologist, QS founding member, and pioneering self-experimentalist—gathered to honor his life and legacy. Seated in a biology lecture hall at UC Berkeley, fellow scientists (both citizen and academic) spoke about their shared experimental lives. "He had skin in the game" went a refrain that echoed throughout. Epistemic debate—around big data and the *n of 1*—mingled with tears. Seth often talked about using self-experimentation to generate ideas for further research. Sometimes it was the only way to test out certain hypotheses or ask questions of personal relevance. His experiments, collaborations, and his prolific and loyally followed blog also spoke to his passion for curiosity. He elevated the smallest, most personal observations into data. Unlike "blind sight" objectivity (Daston 1992), where the subject is a hindrance to truth, Seth's "skin in the game" made him more trustworthy and marked him as anti-establishment. He was memorialized by others who also live life experimentally, who make the everyday amenable to scientific inquiry, and serve as examples of what I call *Homo experimentus*.

Others in the QS community push for self-experimentation as normative science. Mark Drangsholt has made the case for single case crossover research design—EBM-speak for *n of 1*. This *n of 1* spans the EBM hierarchy, elevating the case report into a quasi-controlled study. The legibility of "single case crossover design" to traditional EBM remains to be determined. The difficulty in translating *n of 1* to EBM perhaps reflects its history, where standardization, reproducibility, scale, and cost containment underpinned its development. While Mark presents his *n of 1* arrhythmia tracking at QS meetings, the "single case crossover design" is presented in scientific settings, fitting into the hierarchy. This *n of 1* appears as a boundary object (Star and Griesemer 1989), translating across multiple forms of objectivity and moral economies of science.

Self-tracking for self-care can also lead to a way out of the silos—the "gravity wells"—that limit medical categorization. For some, medical mysteries lead to diagnostic odysseys, for others self-tracking trouble shoots symptoms beyond simplistic pharmacological regimens. Both use the *n of 1* for self-efficacy. QS organizer Anne Wright makes a strong case for the distinction between self- and other-tracking; the former is a way of reclaiming a sense of dignity in the search for answers to personal suffering. Having control over who and what is tracked, for whose ends and on whose terms are all crucial elements to self-tracking, leading toward hope and control in the face of chronic illness. Tracking this way is a technology of the self that operationalizes some of what Annemarie Mol called "the logic of care," which leaves medical measurement open ended to inquiry and the needs of the situation, opposed to logics of (consumer) choice and cure. Some models of tracking for clinical problem solving utilize a coach (rather than a physician) to guide self-discovery. The coach and the self—mirrored in data—provide the relational foundation to this logic of care. Unlike popular considerations of QS, this *n of 1* is not (only) rooted in consuming dHealth technologies (Mol's "logic of choice"). Enabling a different form of medical knowledge production, it refuses the logics of scale, aggregation, and standardization. Like feminist self-helpers, this *n of 1* "diagnosed and redirected the exercise of power as it moved through technical practices that invested ... health with new political dispositions" (Murphy 2012, 32). Tracking ones own biometrics and symptoms with devices or simple spreadsheets, reflecting on them with coaches and data visualization tools[23] redirect the clinical gaze, and invest it in self-determination.

This paraclinical work—asserting the ability to derive valid and useful knowledge from personally collected data—dovetails with participatory medicine's (DeBronkart 2013) clarion call, "give me my DAM data!" (DAM is "data about me"). Agitation over health data—who collects them, how and when they are used and accessed, where they are stored—points to the epistemic, affective, and political stakes contained in this *n of 1*.

The *n of 1* as diversely practiced in QS (a small sampling of which is presented here) consists of a social field where the moral economies of science and medicine are at play. To start, it enables a reassertion of subjectivity and affective attachments in knowledge production, and performs a political operation by relocating the site and terms of clinical tracking. The *n of 1* can also make space for what remains outside of or exceeds the narrow clinical frame, where diagnostic categories, paradigms, and hierarchies of evidence (from the SOAP note to EBM) reign. Here, I think of chronic disease patients I have met who tracked to "hack" their fatigue or seemingly idiosyncratic flares—concerns that barely make the cut in a short office visit with their doctor. Their data round out the portrait.[24] Next, I consider how *n of 1* operates as narrative, reframing the challenges of humanistic medicine.

## Living the Data Stream: *n of 1* as Deep Data

After a long walk where Karen detailed the second part of her long saga caring for her sick child, reorienting her entire world, and the worlds of the hospital around her and her home, we sat to dinner. There was never a strict separation of our formal oral history interviews from the informal time we spent together in and around their home, where traces of their medical home and their lost daughter remain. "This was her hospital, sanctuary, and a home!" she told me late one evening. They are there in the remaining prayer flags that adorn the walls, the logs that tracked her daughter's life and health (from symptoms to diaper changes), and herbal remedies like "Liver Failure Tea" that still fill the cabinets. "It's all data, to me."

Author's Field Note (August 2014)

In the 1990s, physician-humanists like Rita Charon promoted the use of the medical humanities and narrative medicine in medical schools (2001). Both patient and doctor narratives—in the form of writing exercises—are used to palliate the rough training, long hours, emotional and physical burnout, and desensitization that were seen to be dehumanizing patient and doctor alike. The turn to narrative was also a response to ascendant technomedicine, which can center care on diagnostics and machines instead of people. Competent scientific management, Charon argued, cannot enable a physician to help patients make meaning out of suffering. Narrative medicine encourages trainees to understand why stories and lifeworlds matter to healing. Relatedly, medical anthropologists have also asserted the importance of narrative to the experience of suffering and healing, aspects that are left out by biomedicine's technological, pharmaceutical, or surgical interventions. Narrative is part of therapeutic practices, woven into the delivery of a prescription, prognostication, or medical education.[25]

These forms of rehabilitating clinical relationships and care sometimes oppose what is human (narrative as experience) to what is techno-scientific (probing, fragmenting data). However, when we pay close attention to the *n of 1*, we hear how data and narrative are sutured together, recuperating aspects of human and patient experience. When a tracker projected a graph of her symptoms onto the big screen at the Quantified Self conference, she implored us to remember, "It's personal!" In a twist of the clinical gaze that uses technologies to ostensibly fragment, reduce, and alienate patients from their own illness experiences (cf. Taussig 1980), self-quantifying domesticates clinical perception and potentially recuperates narrative, time, and experience. This depends, of course, on the kind of engagement, context, and respect for the affective entanglements of science.

In QS, personal data may function to extend the narrative, as a scaffolding or medium for narrativizing experience. "It's all data to me" expresses the notion that the *n of 1* can be used to gather personal experience, remnants of the past, memorializations of space and time as worthy of being counted. Karen is not trying to aggregate or calculate for the purpose of scientific argument, or for "presenting" to the doctor a "good history."[26] Her tracking was at home, where she created an in-home care space for her terminally ill daughter, displacing the locus of care from the hospital, pulling together a huge community of caregivers—from nurses to neighbors—into their orbit. The few times they felt they had go to the hospital—acute crises—they snuck in their own food for her feeding tube (contraband in the hospital, so the staff were not allowed to administer it), with the staff sometimes in collusion with these small acts of resistance. While not all aspects of their paraclinical care entailed data collection, self- (or kin- in this case) tracking of symptoms, medicines, and diaper changes was a constituent part of their home as both clinic and sanctuary. The data logs, Karen explained, were also an entry point for those who wanted to join and help out—it gave them something to do, marking and tracing not just the numbers, but their attentiveness, presence, and care. Nurses visited the home, lingering longer than they should. A neighbor, a trained scientist, managed the tracking logs. Others planted a garden of therapeutic herbs alongside the house. Their cosmopolitan therapeutics also included experimental pharmaceuticals, which they tracked alongside other masses of her daughter's data.

I call the way they lived the data stream *deep data*. Partly a subtype of big data (Nafus and Sherman 2014), the *n of 1* enables a proliferation of personal data, aided by technologies of the clinic, charting, imaging, or biometrics. The bigness of the data is both probing and fine-grained—the "high-def human." The data are extended and deepened by social stakes hinged to it and its collection. Data are collected, recollected, and marks time, presence, and events on the scale of the everyday. As the fruit of the paraclinical, deep data knits together in productive tension what is often mistakenly opposed: objectifying calculation of clinical gazes and navigating personal and social meaning.[27]

As part of paraclinical care, the *n of 1* situates oneself in one's own life, attending to its specificity. For self-trackers of chronic disease this function is especially important for participating in a medical system that only has so much bandwidth to take in the complexities of living with chronic disease, let alone the context of family or community. The *n of 1* might provide a way to stare back at a clinical gaze whose surveillance probes much but actually sees very little.[28] While the clinical gaze is accused of being panoptic or omnipresent (biomedicalization), the *n of 1* points to its blind spots, to what is unseen or distorted.

## Coda: Caring in Real Time

In another auto-ethnographic account, Janelle Taylor (2008) describes caring for her mother with dementia, and the nagging question asked by many around her: "Does she recognize you?" This question frustrated Taylor because it made her mother's loss of herself as tantamount to the inability to have a caring relationship. It assumed that caring for and about someone requires selves that are stable, coherent, and cognitively situated in the world. She describes, instead, care that is immanent in her mother's seemingly idiosyncratic gestures, habits, and detours into memory—a logic that does not require an idea of personhood that requires recognition. Rather, she urges us to "start looking more at how 'selfhood' is distributed among networks, sustained by supportive environments, emergent within practices of care." This self recalls the *dividual*,[29] a distributed subject, held together by relationships and attachments of care.

My mother's death didn't have this potential. The permanently comatose—the total absence of recognition—lacks biomedical definitions of selfhood. Strangely, she may have qualified for quantified selfhood, not only because of her pixelation and saturation with data, but because of the ways that data tethered her to us. When gathered in an ICU pod, we were not "getting the numbers" in the same way as the medical team. Instead, we rode every single up and down; five minutes sometimes felt like an eternity. As she entered a persistent vegetative state the numbers seem duplicitous: they were taking her away from us, they were all that was left. Those experimenting with QS technique reinvest data with new kinds of meaning and forms of subjectivity, where life is not excluded from the data, but breathed into and with it. Perhaps, tending to my mother's numbers was a form of care in real time. Dismissing a grimace or movement as merely neurologically involuntary short-circuited our caring practices. Her personhood was felt in the presence of family and friends, tethered by invisible strands of kinship and vectors of care. Perhaps we just surfed the data stream to hang on.

## Notes

1. I borrow the term "data exhaust" from Chris Dancy, billed as the most quantified man. He imagines data that streams off of us and our personal effects like car exhaust.

2. Whitney Erin Boesel (2013b) has made a useful distinction between "little" qs and "big" QS—the former being the tracking that people engage in (by buying a fitness tracker or being tracked by their phone, for example) without explicitly claiming ties to the Quantified Self community or movement. "Big" QS is the latter. I mostly deal with the latter, although I refer to reference tools that are used in a "little" qs way.

3. Throughout this chapter, I often draw on the analytical lenses of the epistemologist and historian of science Hans-Jörg Rheinberger (1997). His work analyzes the iterative processes of experimentation and experimental systems, how new questions are formulated, and discoveries revealed.

4. A single lead electrocardiogram (EKG) built into a portable iPhone case. See http://www.alivecor.com/home.

5. The paraclinical also borrows from the "para-ethnographic." Developed by anthropologists Douglas Holmes and George Marcus (2008), the para-ethnographic addresses contemporary ethnography of expert communities.

6. Analysts of direct-to-consumer (DTC) genomics examine how glossing these products as "recreational" distracts from and elides their complex clinical and personal medical meanings for users (Bolnick et al. 2007).

7. On the domestication of on particular clinical technology, the pregnancy test, see Childerhose and Macdonald (2013).

8. I take this term "graft" from Rheinberger (1997) who uses Derrida's use of this term to understand how experimental systems generate new knowledge through repetition, differences, and displacement. I think of the paraclinical and QS *n of 1* as a kind of experimental system.

9. The earliest uses of graphs in American clinical medicine began appearing in the early twentieth century, and accompanied not the availability of technology but a change in practice where tests were transformed into monitoring devices, and encouraged by the proliferation of the earliest forms of health information technology: standardized forms.

10. For an account of the impact of EBM on other realms of health care, such as global health and development projects, see Adams (2013).

11. Represented publicly as the life-hacking work of Tim Ferris and Dave Asprey.

12. These issues were discussed at a session at the 2013 Quantified Self Global Conference.

13. Formulated by QS organizer Anne Wright.

14. A practice quite resonant with anthropological inquiry, in which ethnography uses the self as a starting point and tool toward understanding. See Ortner (1995) for one particular articulation of this. Thanks to Dawn Nafus for pointing this out explicitly here.

15. Inspired here by the work of Anna Tsing (2005) on the productive capacities of frontiers.

16. On promises and pitfalls of big data medicine, see Neff (2013); boyd and Crawford (2012).

17. The human genome has also been characterized this way, an information-rich, natural, and collective resource. For example of deCODE in Iceland, see Winickoff (2006).

18. For example, a presentation by a "Quant-friendly Doctor" tracks with patients, yet resolutely keeps their data out of their electronic health record.

19. Of note: "Insight" is the name of a data analytics tool created and sold by the electronic medical record company, Practice Fusion. In data science, insights perhaps reflect the provisional nature of results from this kind of research. Unlike truth, the object of experimental science, "insight" is the kind of knowledge produced in a modulating system, where information is gathered and processed in "real time"; see https://insight.practicefusion.com/, accessed August 31, 2015.

20. Exemplified by dHealth tools and studies such as the Health eHeart Study, dubbed the digital Framingham Study, where participants' dHealth devices (pedometers, scales, blood pressure cuffs, AliveCors) are synced to the study's cloud servers, so that you may take care of yourself through self-tracking while simultaneously merging your numbers to a larger dataset. The Framingham Study was a prospective cohort study. "Cohort" may be obsolete now as *n of 1* data streams flow into the open-ended set.

21. See Daston and Galison (2010).

22. Some QS projects connect to civic projects such as using citizen scientists to gather data on local pollution: for example, Carnegie Mellon University's CREATE Lab's water-quality project, http://www.cmucreatelab.org/projects/Water_Quality_Monitoring/pages/CATTFish(accessed August 15, 2015). However, the status of politics (small p) is a point of contention. There was an attempt to address social structures and politics at one panel at the 2014 Quantified Self European Conference. Instead, the conversation became tense when a few members of the audience felt condescended to, and claimed that QS was about them working on themselves.

23. Like the CREATE lab's Fluxtream tool: https://fluxtream.org/.

24. Data as portrait is explored in QS by the artists who present their work at QS events, translating data into artistic artifacts or portraits. See the work of Laurie Frick, for example, who just completed a Kickstarter campaign to make a phone application to help people turn their data into art: https://www.kickstarter.com/projects/lauriefrick/frickbits-your-data-is-now-art-on-your-iphone(accessed August 15, 2015).

25. For a selection see Del Vecchio Good et al. (1994); Mattingly (1994); Kohn (2000); Mattingly and Garro (2000); Good and Good (2000).

26. In the clinical context, and told to us in training, patients are often praised or admonished (not in front of them) as being either "good or reliable historians" or "bad historians" of their own illness experiences.

27. This can also be read as the convergence of the Foucauldian idea that modern power operates by our using expertise to know ourselves intimately. However, in QS the use of the *n of 1* offers a different relationship to expertise, one where it is undermined in the course of creating new epistemologies of medicine and the self.

28. Thanks to Dawn Nafus for helping to articulate this.

29. For more on Marilyn Strathern's *dividual*, see Smith (2012).

## References


Adams, Vincanne. 2013. "Evidence-based global public health." In *When People Come First*, ed. J. Biehl and A. Petryna, 54–90. Princeton: Princeton University Press.

Armstrong, David. 1995. "The Rise of Surveillance Medicine." *Sociology of Health & Illness* 17 (3): 393–405.

Beck, Ulrich. 1992. *Risk Society: Towards a New Modernity*. London: Sage Publications.

Berg, M. 1995. "Turning a Practice into a Science: Reconceptualizing Postwar Medical Practice." *Social Studies of Science* 25 (3): 437–476.

Berg, M. 2004. "Embodying the Patient: Records and Bodies in Early 20th-Century US Medical Practice." *Body & Society* 10 (2–3) (June 1): 13–41.

Boesel, Whitney Erin. 2013a. "Data Occupations." *The New Inquiry* (November 25). http://thenewinquiry.com/essays/data-occupations/. Accessed August 18, 2015.

Boesel, Whtiney Erin. 2013b. "What is the Quantified Self Now?" http://thesocietypages.org/cyborgology/2013/05/22/what-is-the-quantified-self-now/. Accessed August 18, 2015.

Bolnick, Deborah, Duana Fullwiley, Troy Duster, Richard S. Cooper, Joan H. Fujimura, Jonathan Kahn, Jay S. Kaufman, et al. 2007. "Genetics. The Science and Business of Genetic Ancestry Testing." *Science* 318 (5849) (October 19): 399–400.

boyd, Danah, and Kate Crawford. 2012. "Critical Questions for Big Data." *Information Communication and Society* 15 (5): 662–679.

Castel, Robert. 1991. "From Dangerousness to Risk." In *The Foucault Effect: Studies in Governmentality*, ed. Graham Burchell, Colin Gordon, and Peter Miller, 281–298. Chicago: University of Chicago Press.

Charon, Rita. 2001. "Narrative Medicine: A Model for Empathy, Reflection, Profession, and Trust." *Journal of the American Medical Association* 286 (15): 1897–1902.

Childerhose, Janet E., and Margaret E. Macdonald. 2013. "Health Consumption as Work: The Home Pregnancy Test as a Domesticated Health Tool." *Social Science & Medicine* 86 (June): 1–8.

Clarke, Adele E, Janet K. Shim, Laura Mamo, Jennifer Ruth Fosket, and R. Jennifer. 2003. "Biomedicalization: Technoscientific Transformations of Health, Illness, and U.S. Biomedicine." *American Sociological Review* 68 (2): 161–194.

Cohen, Lawrence. 2004. "Operability, Bioavailability, and Exception." In *Global Assemblages: Technology, Politics, and Ethics as Anthropological Problems*, ed. Aihwa Ong and Stephen J. Collier, 79–90. London: Blackwell Publishing.

Daston, L. 1992. "Objectivity and the Escape from Perspective." *Social Studies of Science* 22 (4) (November 1): 597–618.

Daston, Lorraine, and Peter Galison. 2010. *Objectivity*. New York: Zone Books.

DeBronkart, e-Patient Dave. 2013. *Let Patients Help!: A Patient Engagement Handbook*. Seattle: CreateSpace Independent Publishing Platform.

Deleuze, G. 1992. "Postscript on the Societies of Control." *October* 59: 3–7.

Del Vecchio Good, Mary-Jo, Tseunetsugu Munakata, Yasuki Kobayashi, Cheryl Mattingly, and Byron J. Good. 1994. "Oncology and Narrative Time." *Social Science & Medicine* 38 (6): 855–862.

Dumit, Joseph. 2003. *Picturing Personhood*. Princeton, NJ: Princeton University Press.

Dumit, Joseph. 2010. "Inter-Pill-Ation and the Instrumentalization of Compliance." *Anthropology & Medicine* 17 (2): 245–247.

Dumit, Joseph. 2012a. *Drugs for Life: How Pharmaceutical Companies Define Our Health*. Durham, NC: Duke University Press.

Dumit, Joseph. 2012b. "Prescription Maximization and the Accumulation of Surplus Health in the Pharmaceutical Industry: The_BioMarx_Experiment." In *Lively Capital*, ed. Kaushik Sunder Rajan, 45–92. Durham, NC: Duke University Press.

Foucault, Michel. 1973. *The Birth of the Clinic*. New York: Vintage Books.

Foucault, Michel. 1986. *The Care of the Self*. vol. 3. History of Sexuality. New York: Vintage Books.

Foucault, Michel. 2004. *The Birth of Biopolitics: Lectures at the College de France, 1978–1979*, eds. Michel Senellart, Arnold I. Davidson, Alessandro Fontana, Francois Ewald, and Graham Burchell. New York: Palgrave.

Gifford, Sandra M. 1986. "The Meaning of Lumps: A Case Study of the Ambiguities of Risk." In *Anthropology and Epidemiology: Interdisciplinary Approaches to the Study of Health and Disease,* ed. Craig Robert Janes, Ron Stall, and Sandra M. Gifford, 213–246. Nowell, MA: Kluwer Academic Publishers.

Good, Byron J., and Mary-Jo Delvecchio Good. 2000. "'Fiction' and 'Historicity' in Doctor's Stories: Social and Narrative Dimensions of Learning Medicine." In *Narrative and the Cultural Construction of Illness and Healing*, ed. Cheryl Mattingly and L. C. Garro, 50–69. Berkeley: University of California Press.

Gordon, Deborah. 1988. "Tenacious Assumptions in Western Medicine." In *Biomedicine Examined*, ed. Margaret Lock and Deborah Gordon, 19–56. Dordrecht: Kluwer Academic Publishers.

Greene, Jeremy. 2008. *Prescribing by Numbers: Drugs and the Definition of Disease*. Baltimore: Johns Hopkins University Press.

Hey, Tony, Stewart Tansley, and Kristin Tolle, eds. 2009. *The Fourth Paradigm: Data-Intensive Scientific Discovery*. Redmond, WA: Microsoft Research.

Holmes, Douglas R., and George E. Marcus. 2008. "Collaboration Today and the Re-Imagination of the Classic Scene of Fieldwork Encounter." *Collaborative Anthropologies* 1: 81–101.

Howell, Joel D. 1995. *Technology in the Hospital*. Baltimore: Johns Hopkins University Press.

Koenig, Barbara A. 1988. "The Technological Imperative in Medical Practice: The Social Creation of a 'Routine' Treatment." In *Biomedicine Examined,* ed. Margaret Lock and Deborah Gordon, 465–496. Dordrecht: Kluwer Academic Publishers.

Kohn, Abigail. 2000. "'Imperfect Angels': Narrative 'Emplotment' in the Medical Management of Children with Craniofacial Anomalies." *Medical Anthropology* 14 (2): 202–223.

Mattingly, Cheryl. 1994. "The Concept of Therapeutic 'Emplotment.'" *Social Science & Medicine* 38 (6): 811–822.

Mattingly, Cheryl, and Linda C. Garro. 2000. *Narrative and the Cultural Construction of Illness and Healing*, ed. Cheryl Mattingly and Linda C. Garro. Berkeley: University of California Press.

Mol, Annemarie. 2002. *The Body Multiple*. Durham, NC: Duke University Press.

Murphy, Michelle. 2012. *Seizing the Means of Reproduction: Entanglements of Feminism, Health, and Technoscience*. vol. 26. Durham, NC: Duke University Press.

Nafus, Dawn, and Jamie Sherman. 2014. "This One Does Not Go Up To Eleven: Quantified Self Movement as an Alternative Big Data Practice." *International Journal of Communication*, 8 (11): 1784–1794.

Neff, Gina. 2013. "Why Big Data Won't Cure Us." *Big Data* 1 (3): 117–123.

Ortner, Sherry B. 1995. "Resistance and the Problem of Ethnographic Refusal." *Society for Comparative Study of Society and History* 37 (1): 173–193.

Ostherr, Kirsten. 2013. *Medical Visions: Producing the Patient Through Film, Television, and Imaging Technologies*. Oxford: Oxford University Press.

Petersen, Allan R, and Deborah Lupton. 1996. *The New Public Health: Health and Self in the Age of Risk*. London: Sage Publications.

Rheinberger, Hans- Jörg. 1997. *Toward a History of Epistemic Things: Synthesizing Proteins in the Test Tube*. Palo Alto, CA: Stanford University Press.

Robert Wood Johnson Foundation. 2014. "Personal Data for the Public Good." http://www.rwjf.org/content/dam/farm/reports/reports/2014/rwjf411080. Accessed August 18, 2015.

Rose, Nikolas. 2007. *The Politics of Life Itself: Biomedicine, Power, and Subjectivity in the Twenty-First Century*. Princeton, NJ: Princeton University Press.

Saunders, Barry F. 2010. *CT Suite: The Work of Diagnosis in the Age of Noninvasive Cutting*. Durham, NC: Duke University Press.

Sinclair, Simon. 2004. "Evidence-Based Medicine: A New Ritual in Medical Teaching." *British Medical Bulletin* 69 (January): 179–196.

Smith, Karl. 2012. "From Dividual and Individual Selves to Porous Subjects." *Australian Journal of Anthropology* 23 (1): 50–64.

Star, Susan Leigh, and James R. Griesemer. 1989. "Institutional Ecology, 'Translations' and Boundary Objects: Amateurs and Professionals in Berkeley's Museum of Vertebrate Zoology, 1907–39." *Social Studies of Science* 19 (3): 387–420.

Sunder Rajan, Kaushik. 2005. "Subjects of Speculation: Emergent Life Sciences and Market Logics in the United States and India." *American Anthropologist* 107 (1): 19–30.

Sunder Rajan, Kaushik. 2006. *Biocapital: The Constitution of Postgenomic Life*. Durham, NC: Duke University Press.

Taussig, Michael T. 1980. "Reification and the Consciousness of the Patient." *Social Science and Medicine. Medical Anthropology* 14B (1): 3–13.

Taylor, Janelle S. 2008. "On Recognition, Caring, and Dementia." *Medical Anthropology Quarterly* 22 (4): 313–335.

Timmermans, S., and M. Berg. 1997. "Standardization in Action: Achieving Local Universality through Medical Protocols." *Social Studies of Science* 27 (2) (April 1): 273–305.

Timmermans, Stefan, and Marc Berg. 2003. *The Gold Standard: The Challenge of Evidence-Based Medicine and Standardization in Health Care*. Philadelphia: Temple University Press.

Topol, Eric J. 2012. *The Creative Destruction of Medicine: How the Digital Revolution Will Create Better Health Care*. New York: Basic Books.

Tsing, Anna Lowenhaupt. 2005. *Friction: An Ethnography of Global Connection*. Princeton, NJ: Princeton University Press.

Whitmarsh, Ian. 2013. "The Ascetic Subject of Compliance: The Turn to Chronic Diseases in Global Health." In *When People Come First: Critical Studies in Global Health*, ed. Joao Biehl and Adriana Petryna, 302–324.Princeton, NJ: Princeton University Press.

Winickoff, David E. 2006. "Genome and Nation: Iceland's Heath Sector Database and Its Legacy." *Innovations: Technology, Governance, Globalization* 1 (2): 80–105.

# 8

# Consumer Health Innovation Opportunities and Privacy Challenges: A View from the Trenches

Rajiv Mehta

What is the potential for disruption in consumer health technologies? How should we address the challenges of privacy in a world aflow in personal health data? As I read the chapters in part II, and contemplated new ideas and new perspectives, my response was strongly influenced by my own experiences. Over the past twenty-five years, almost every product or business I have worked on, for large companies such as Apple and Symbol and numerous startups, has fit the model of disruptive innovation. For much of the past decade my focus has been on consumer health: on how people take care of themselves and their families; on how they view and fit these activities in the context of their lives; on the challenges they face in doing what they would like to do; and on technologies, products, and services that could make their activities both easier and more effective.

## The Challenge of Open Spaces for Disruptive Consumer Health Technologies

Disruptive innovation implies unorthodox, non-mainstream thinking. In health innovation, however, most investors and media, as well as the general public, expect leadership, or at least involvement, by the health-care establishment. I believe that a fundamental difficulty in disruptive consumer health innovation stems from the lack of health spaces willingly ignored by the medical establishment, and from the public's acceptance of the hegemony of the establishment on things even tangentially related to health.

The iPhone comes with a set of well-designed productivity apps, and there are many alternatives for purchase. Consumers do not inquire whether the developers included licensed productivity experts on their teams; do not look for approvals by productivity associations; and do not expect proof of "outcomes" (e.g., healthier business profits). Instead, consumers choose based on price, vendor reputation, reviews, recommendations, and the vendor-provided description. Though many people use these tools for health management (e.g., putting doctor appointments or medication reminders in calendars), there is no expectation of FDA reviews or AMA approval. And no one expects that health insurance will pay for the apps.

My own efforts have met with very different expectations. Over the past few years I have developed a series of apps (Zume Life, then Tonic, then Unfrazzle) that are essentially productivity apps, but tailored to help the user remember and keep track of care activities (the things they do to take care of themselves and other family members). For example, care activities can involve schedule rhythms ("every 3rd week on Monday and Tuesday at 7am and 5pm") that normal productivity apps are not designed for. Unlike the products and services described in chapter 6 by Fiore-Gartland and Neff, these apps provide absolutely no medical advice or analysis. They are essentially calendars-cum-notebooks. However, because these apps are for care activities, which implies a health issue, investors, reviewers, health professionals, and often even consumers themselves, have expectations that health professionals have been involved, that health outcomes have been proven through clinical studies, that health providers will prescribe the app to their patients, and so on.

In fact, most consumer care (self-care and family caregiving) has little to do with professional medicine. The situation is admittedly confusing, as there is simultaneously more and less medicine-in-the-home than commonly perceived. On the one hand, consumer care today involves many more medical and nursing tasks than ever before, as described in *Home Alone*.[1] On the other hand, it is also true, as noted by Greenfield in chapter 7 and also described in the report *Catalyzing Technology to Support Family Caregiving*,[2] that the vast majority of care tasks are nonmedical.

In chapter 6, Fiore-Gartland and Neff probe the potential for and challenges of "disruptive innovation" in health and wellness technologies. They note that definitions and framing matter enormously, to both expectations and outcomes. As they note, it is "discourses about industry disruption"—how the concept of disruption is discussed in the popular/business media, rather than how it is described in the innovation academic literature—that sets expectations and impacts funding and other business decisions. While there is a lot of talk about how technology is going to disrupt the health market, actual disruption seems slow in coming.

As chapter 6 describes, citing the writing of Clayton Christensen and others, in business and technology academia "disruptive innovation" implies a business area that begins by new companies addressing markets that at the time are poorly served, and often actively ignored, by the entrenched players. The "disruption" occurs later, often much later, if and when the "low-end" products get "good enough" for mainstream needs. By then it is often too late for the original entrenched players to react strongly, and the new players are able to hold onto their market positions. Not all, in fact very few, of the efforts to address unserved markets end up disrupting the major markets. As innovation research has shown, the entrenched players are usually quite aware of the ignored markets, and have chosen to ignore them for good reasons. If others want to waste their resources trying to address such markets, the entrenched players are happy to allow them do so. This allowance is critical. It opens the door to possible, though rare, disruptive innovation.

As a personal experience, I led Apple's entry into the digital camera market, launching the QuickTake 100 in 1994. It got a lot of attention, most of the market share, and sparked the digital camera revolution. In today's terms, the QuickTake took very poor images. Even for its time, the QuickTake's image quality was poor, far inferior to even the worst, film-based disposable cameras. However, Apple felt that there was a market for a camera that made picture taking for computer use very easy and quick, even with barely good-enough image quality. The entrenched photography players could see no business value in such a low-quality product. The Apple team sometimes faced polite ridicule as we tried to meet with dominant industry players as potential business and technology partners. One major player would not even take a meeting, apparently feeling the idea was so absurd that it was not worth the time to discuss. Another urged us toward a $10,000 digital camera that could take pictures "better than film" though we kept asking for something "under $300." Finally Kodak, whose executives would not countenance getting into such a market themselves, accepted a contract because its technology team wanted at least a buyer for their components. The disruptive innovator, in this case Apple, was possible because the entrenched players chose to ignore the market. They did not believe there was a significant-enough market to be worth their attention, and they were not bothered if another company tried to address such a market.

For innovators hoping to disrupt health, a fundamental challenge is that the entrenched players fiercely guard and constantly expand the space they consider to be their domain. Even if the entrenched players will not serve a need themselves, they insist on being the gatekeepers, the voices of authority, and will fight to disallow new entrants space for innovation, as has happened to 23andMe.

"The dream of reason did not take power into account." So begins Paul Starr's Pulitzer Prize winning history of American medicine, *The Social Transformation of American Medicine*.[3] Starr notes that although we generally believe that medicine has advanced through scientific progress, power-politics has played a significant role. "But reason is no abstract force pushing inexorably toward greater freedom at the end of history. Its forms and uses are determined by the narrower purposes of men and women; their interests and ideals shape even what counts as knowledge. … In America, no one group has held so dominant a position in this new world of rationality and power as has the medical profession." The American medical profession, the entrenched players in American health, fought hard to achieve their hegemony. Today the medical profession no longer has to fight alone. Society has generally come to accept members of the medical establishment as the ultimate authority on anything related to health, and expect them to wield such authority. In practice, this boils down to no health innovation without the explicit involvement and approval of the entrenched players, and hence no opportunity for disruptive innovation.

When entrenched players lead, what one gets is almost always "sustaining innovation." These are improvements that serve existing markets (through better, faster, cheaper products) and can be sold through existing value networks. Mostly these innovations provide incremental improvements (evolutionary), though sometimes they provide huge leaps forward (revolutionary). Sustaining innovations do not change markets, they are not disruptive.

Though my own consumer-centric health-related products (Zume Life, Tonic, and Unfrazzle) are essentially productivity tools, provide no medical advice, and rely on no medical science, most people expect that these products have been developed with the oversight of medical experts, should be "prescribed" by doctors, and should be paid for through traditional health-care payment models. The public expects and supports the hegemony of the health-care establishment. Unfortunately, due to a messy brew of health-care organizational silos, legal concerns, and mindsets about patients, such consumer-centric products are of low interest to the health-care establishment. The sustaining innovation equivalents of my products are "adherence" apps (sometimes focused on medications, sometimes focused on activities associated with a specific disease). Unfortunately, such products do not fully serve consumer's care management needs.[4] Basically here is a market need that is poorly served by the establishment, but not easily addressable by players outside the establishment.

Imagine if the consumer computer industry had been hobbled by such hegemony. Imagine if in the 1970s IBM had been perceived as the ultimate authority on computing, that its okay was required before computing technologies could be used by the untrained public. Would white-coated professionals have argued that putting such power into consumer hands was dangerous, that people could do themselves harm by making plans based on miscalculations? Would they have argued that it was best to leave it to them (IBM), but that they unfortunately would not be able to address consumer demands unless someone was willing to pay them their regular high-priced fees for educating the public or for developing such low-end products? Then the innovators in the Homebrew Computer Club[5] might not have had much impact, and the Apple II would likely not have sparked the personal computing revolution. Advocates of personal computing would have been forced to prove that consumers would use such power responsibly, that they would not cause harm to themselves or others, that they would go through full training prior to using such technologies, and that they would always carefully follow and not veer from expert directions. Change would have been much, much slower.

If no aspect of health is viewed as beyond the purview of existing health care, is the construct of "disruptive innovation" inappropriate for the sector of health? I am optimistic that innovation will find a way. The problem may be in the language, in the use of words like "health" and "care." For example, there is in fact lots of innovation happening in fields such as exercise, fitness, yoga, meditation, diet, and sleep—all critical to good health—that are unconstrained by expectations of health-care establishment leadership. With large companies like Apple, and thousands of entrepreneurs worldwide, new products will find their way to market, and will steadily encroach on "health" and "care." The modern equivalents of the Homebrew Computer Club, such as the Quantified Self movement, are prying open spaces where approvals by the health-care establishment are not required.

## User-Managed Controls Cannot Be the Solution to the Privacy Problem

Nissenbaum and Patterson in chapter 5 break down the technologies, information flows, and users of personal data. In laying out taxonomies and frameworks for analysis they also make it easier to see the complexity of the privacy problem. My own effort to provide consumers with tools to manage privacy in a small, and perhaps the easiest, setting—among close family members—highlights the challenge. In my experience, such privacy-control tools are necessary but far from sufficient, not very usable in practice, and difficult to justify as a business decision.

In their chapter, Patterson and Nissenbaum provide some important history, taking us back to an earlier time of increased privacy concerns, to the 1890 *Harvard Law Review* article by Samuel Warren and Louis Brandeis advocating for the right "to be left alone" based on their concerns about the decrease in privacy resulting from recent innovations in photography and publishing. These innovations made the capture and distribution of personal information much easier. Warren and Brandeis's recommendations focused on tort law, arguing that those who misuse private data should have to pay for the consequences of their actions, rather than advocating for direct limitations on photography or printing. They placed the burden on users of the photographs to do so properly, not on the photographed subjects to clearly stipulate if, how, and when their photographs could be taken or used. The same line of thinking today, given the complexity of the personal data privacy problem, presumably leads to placing the burden on users of private data to do so properly, and be liable for any harm they cause, and not on individuals to clearly stipulate if, how, and when their data can be gathered or used.

The authors make a valuable point about privacy concerns being contextual. Who has our information, and under what circumstances, matters a great deal. Employers, product manufacturers, health-care professionals, and many others interested in making use of personal data may not always place top priority on the person's best interests. It is also clear that for an average person, making a well-considered decision to share private data, carefully weighing the pros and cons, may be very difficult, at the very least time consuming, and quite often beyond that person's capabilities. Following Warren and Brandeis's recommendation, rather than place the burden on individuals to state when and how their data can be used, it would be best if there was a legal framework that penalized the users of personal biosensor data for any harm caused to those persons.

The authors observe that designers must make technical architecture decisions that affect how much control users have over where data go, and therefore it is incumbent upon designers to have a better understanding of where people would want to be able to constrain the circulation of data. They state, "If we want architecture to embody these constraints, we must first know what the constraints are, and we should have the means of holding designers accountable for their design choices." We must also, however, recognize the limits of design; some things are better managed outside the product.

No matter how good the technical architecture and interface design of privacy controls, such controls place significant burdens on users to understand who might use their data, how the data might be used, and potential consequences. As even experts cannot properly foresee all potential major consequences, it seems unreasonable to expect an average consumer to make a well-thought-out decision regarding the use of her data by businesses, health institutions, and so on. Therefore consumer tools for privacy controls may have little practical value. An exception is within "the home," the network of close family and friends. In this context the user may have strong preferences regarding data sharing, and likely knows the individuals and social dynamics better than any outside expert.

Designing and developing such privacy controls and appropriate interfaces is difficult. As one example, the Unfrazzle[6] app allows a user to get reminders for and make notes about all care-related activities that he is responsible for, whether for his own well-being or for others he cares for. The user can also allow other family members and friends to view or modify his entries, make entries on his behalf, and even to make fundamental changes to his regimen (his list of activities, schedules, etc.). The user has extremely fine-grained control over which activities are accessible to which family members and at what level (view-only, modify, etc.), and such permissions can be changed by the user at any time. The downside of all this flexibility and control is that the user needs to think carefully about family members before making data-sharing decisions, and to modify these decisions as relationships evolve. Fortunately, there are default settings that work well under most circumstances. The irony is that creating this user control system was a lot of work, and in practice is hardly ever used. Product developers rightly will spend far more time on features that users want and use, than on those such as these privacy controls that are almost never used. I still believe that such controls must be developed, despite their difficulty, for those unplannable circumstances when the user absolutely needs them, but given the very high opportunity cost of providing such controls developers must be careful to limit the controls to the minimum possible.

As another example, consider the privacy controls provided by Apple, a company with the resources, technology skills, and design acumen to do a very good job. As they bluntly note on their privacy website[7] (as of this writing, Fall 2014), their business does not rely on leveraging users' private data, and so their decisions to provide users control are not hamstrung by other business considerations. In a section "Privacy Built In," Apple describes the things their products do automatically to minimize privacy breaches, such as randomly changing a device's MAC address so that it cannot be easily tracked across Wi-Fi networks. Apple also provides numerous user controls described in a section "Manage Your Privacy"—a long list presented beautifully and explained clearly. And yet, my impression is that few users (including myself) will be able to fully understand all the options and use them wisely.

Patterson and Nissenbaum think about new technology as changing currently existing information flows. It seems to me that, regarding data privacy, we are tackling not new philosophical issues but rather unsettled ones, previously kept at bay through practical considerations. When music was sold on delicate wax cylinders, one didn't have to deeply explore philosophical questions about the actual limits of "personal use" regarding copying. When health information was handwritten in a doctor's notebook, one didn't have to worry too much about who else would look at it. By removing the practical difficulties, new technologies are forcing us to confront difficult philosophical questions. The burden for answering should not be on the shoulders of each individual consumer. As recommended by Warren and Brandeis we must find viable policy solutions instead.

## Designing for Consumer Needs

So, what is the potential for disruption in consumer health technologies? I believe the potential is enormous. Consumers have significant, unaddressed (or very poorly addressed) needs, which have a huge, well-known negative impact on their own physical and mental health and finances, in addition to major societal costs. I believe that those who aspire to disrupt the consumer health industry, to develop innovations to help consumers achieve their health-related goals, and do so in ways that protect their privacy, will be more successful if they design for people[8] (consumers) rather than designing for "patients," if they frame the issue in a consumer rather than a health-care perspective.

## Notes

1. Susan Reinhard, Carol Levine, and Sarah Samis, *Home Alone: Family Caregivers Providing Complex Chronic Care.* AARP Public Policy Institute/United Hospital Fund, October 2012, http://www.uhfnyc.org/publications/880853, accessed August 31, 2015.

2. Richard Adler and Rajiv Mehta, "Catalyzing Technology to Support Family Caregiving," National Alliance for Caregiving, July 2014, http://bit.ly/caretech14.

3. Paul Starr, *The Social Transformation of American Medicine* (New York: Basic Books, 1982).

4. Rajiv Mehta, "8 Years to the Model T: Zume Life to Unfrazzle, Findings from a Long Strange Trip," presentation at Health Foo, Boston, December 2013, http://youtu.be/sZo0YS3OljA.

5. Paul Freiberger and Michael Swaine, *Fire in the Valley: The Making of the Personal Computer* (Whitbey, Ontario: McGraw-Hill Professional, 1999).

6. http://unfrazzledcare.com/unfrazzle_app/.

7. http://www.apple.com/privacy.

8. Hugh Dubberly, Rajiv Mehta, Shelley Evenson, and Paul Pangaro, "Reframing Health to Embrace Design of Our Own Well-being," *Interactions* 17, no. 3 (2010): 56–63, http://www.dubberly.com/articles/reframing-health.html.

# III

## Seeing Like a Builder

The chapters of part III ask what a biosensor-rich world looks like from the perspective of people who build these technologies, and the social and cultural formations that go alongside them. In some ways, part III picks up on the essential themes articulated earlier in the book—how data renegotiate relations between self and other, how biomedicalization and counter-practices jostle for cultural legitimacy, and how existing institutional forms shape what comes on the market. Part III gives these themes a material grounding that helps us better assess what could, and what should, happen with biosensor data, by helping us see what biosensor creators see through building. When someone approaches biosensing (or any other technical practice for that matter) with an eye toward designing it differently, what she notices is very different from what jumps out when she has her eye on social commentary. By approaching biosensing from this angle, we become sensitized to what is more open to change, what is difficult to shift, and what is surprisingly simple. This angle is particularly valuable for those of us who would like to intervene, whether our interest is in building something ourselves, as the scholars in the chapters of part III have done, or more traditional social science activities such as informing policy change. Some of these chapters underscore the peril of trying to do one independently from the other.

These chapters make clear that building yields surprises from any number of corners. The surprises come once the builder gets into the technical weeds, and finds that unseen complexities make themselves apparent. They also come through the sometimes surprising places where one meets social resistance, or where people use what a creator has built in ways she did not envision. Each chapter approaches surprises in different ways. Estrin and de Paula Hanika (chapter 9) design around what they know they cannot anticipate, thus incorporating flexibility into a system that otherwise could become rigid. Böhlen's chapter (chapter 10) conveys particularly well what it is like to be in the thick of these surprises, and having to change course constantly in response to them. Taylor (chapter 11) dips his toes in data processing in ways designed to provoke alternatives to stable categories currently used in data work. In my own work building data processing software,[1] I too have been struck by precisely how little can be anticipated, and how much one can only really learn by doing. Yet I am also struck by the paradox that emerges when we compare Taylor's and Böhlen's contributions. On the one hand, Böhlen shows us that to build in ways sensitive to the belief systems already in place is to find surprises. On the other hand, when Taylor looks at what is being built today, he largely sees the same old categories and social systems embodied in new technologies. His claim is that it is possible to build something new and not be surprised *enough*. Put together, these two scholars show us that perhaps going beyond "same old categories" invites more uncertainty in already uncertain work. When building something, one has to choose what one is going to hold stable, and what one seeks to change. To build in ways that embody more fundamental social change perhaps requires slower building.

In the pages to come, you will develop a sense of how these surprises unfold. They raise important questions about the relationship between policy and design described in part II. Gregory and Bowker in chapter 12 suggest that policies that govern biosensing technologies cannot be thought about outside the specific technological conditions that bring people and things together, and shape public and private, which, like Day and Lury, they see as an unfixed distinction. This raises an important point. If we agree that privacy is important (even if as necessary fiction—surely there is room to deconstruct the very things we want?), then we must also agree with Patterson and Nissenbaum that some level of due diligence is warranted. But Gregory and Bowker raise the next, equally difficult question: if due diligence cannot be carried out independently from the technology, at what moment in the technical development should such an exercise be undertaken? It seems useless to try if all a technology developer has is the faintest notion of what she wants to create, and it seems too late after millions, or in some cases billions, of dollars have been spent creating it. "In the middle!" is an obvious answer—the one given by privacy-by-design advocates. My own experience in building has led me to believe that this is wise in general, but there is also a certain unhelpful vagueness in the suggestion to build in privacy "along the way." Exactly when and how to rethink a decision, in the context of competing problems to deal with, is not obvious. How elaborately should one trace out all possible scenarios? How do you know it is better to undo expensively built code than to continue with the code you have? If only "the way" were a linear, predictable path! The chapters of part III will offer a sense of what being in the middle is actually like, or could be like, in hopes of offering a ground-level view into the moments when considerations like privacy can (and cannot) be taken into account.

All of the projects presented here are also attempts to do things differently; that is, they are not accounts of straightforward product development that would likely yield more of the same types of products the market now generates. These are technology developers who are extraordinarily careful about the social relationships their technologies make possible. As such, they are well positioned to describe what it is like to live with a box of surprises you have just opened, and now have to deal with. In the Introduction, I suggested that we in the social sciences could help technology developers embrace the possibility that alternative social relations could be built into material worlds, or to use Taylor's phrase, "material worlds that enliven relations rather than flatten them." These changes would be more substantial than the constant stream of "revolutions" declared by Silicon Valley rhetoric. If we are going to ask for such things, then part of the work on our end has to be comprehending when and how we would have builders embrace even more uncertainty than they already work with by necessity. Seeing the uncertainties that builders perceive can support the formulation of design recommendations that can be taken up more easily. It can also inform judgments about when it might be necessary for social scientists to "roll their own," as the software developers like to say, and directly build the things we would like to see in the world. "Rolling our own" requires more skills than those taught in social science departments, but is not that far-fetched. In fact, the 2015 annual meeting of STS scholars hosted demonstrations of software, hardware, and other physical building projects from social science and humanities scholars who build.

In part III we have a diversity of approaches to building. Taylor's contribution could be described as a critical making project, in Matt Ratto's (2011) original sense of building something physical in order to explore a theory or social phenomenon through materials. Here Taylor builds an assemblage of data, and takes nonobvious cuts through it to explore what capacities are being undervalued. In their chapters, Böhlen and Estrin and de Paula Hanika surface the nuances of the social and material world by working their way through it, backing off on what does not work, and elaborating on what does. Building can also be building a team, or building the kinds of constructs or imagery intended to inspire a different material world. Gregory and Bowker have not built a technology per se, but they are included here because they have written with an eye toward intervention, grounded in a particularly sensitive attention to materials.

It has been multiple decades since STS and aligned disciplines began to take materials seriously, having had enough time to recover from the fallacies of technological determinism. The contributors in part III have gone beyond thinking about materials as a theoretical conceit. Some use materials to make their contributions to social scientific knowledge, while others more plainly, and with a good deal of generosity, open up their work so that we in the social sciences might see what they see. The street goes both ways. Building has something to offer the social sciences and humanities, by making objects that are also good to think with. Those disciplines in turn have much to offer those who would reshape the built world. If we are to intervene while technologies are being built rather than attempting to undo them after the fact, seeing with an eye toward building is necessary.

## Note

1. The data processing software is a cloud-based tool called Data Sense. It can be found at www.makesenseofdata.com.

## Reference

Ratto, Matt. 2011. "Critical Making: Conceptual and Material Studies in Technology and Social Life." *Information Society* 27 (4): 252–260.

# 9

# Open mHealth and the Problem of Data Interoperability

Deborah Estrin and Anna de Paula Hanika, with Dawn Nafus

## Editor's Introduction

"Data flows." "Data exhaust." "Seamlessness." "Openness." The words we use to describe data, both popularly and in the social sciences, often imply that data remains comprehensible as it moves around. In part III, we will hear from a range of authors who work directly with the technical systems that shape what people can and cannot do with data. Before we get to those chapters, however, it is useful to have more grounding in the technical aspects of data. There are more steps than we ordinarily assume between "raw" sensor data and data that is helpful for making judgments about a medical condition. To make data legible as it moves from one system to the next is a nontrivial technical challenge, even before we get to the social challenges. To understand what is actually involved, I sat down with Deborah Estrin, a computer scientist at Cornell University and cofounder of Open mHealth,[1] a nonprofit startup that aims to bring clinical meaning to digital health data through an open platform designed for improved interoperability among disparate, heterogeneous data sources. This is not a raw interview transcript. Estrin, de Paula Hanika, and I collaboratively converted our conversation into written commentary.

**DN**: What is Open mHealth?

**DE**: Open mHealth offers a way of describing patient-generated data so that it can be interpretable throughout the health-care system. What does that mean, exactly? Think about how the Internet works. When it was built, there was not one usage people had in mind, but a set of components that worked together in an open and modular way. Those components are things that we use over and over again. You can think about it like Home Depot—you can get components like screws, bolts, and pipes that are standard sizes from different companies and get replacement parts without having to go back to that original company. The Internet was built with standardized interfaces, and that modular architecture is what allowed everything to grow.

Open mHealth is trying to do something similar for data relevant for health care—"relevant" meaning that the person is not necessarily a medical patient, but could be doing health-related things on her own, or capturing data that could be relevant to her health. We are in a situation where mobile phones are changing, wearables are changing, people have new ideas for user engagement, what to measure, etc. Potential types of data don't just include "blood pressure" but "time I spent on social media" or "how much I ate." If you had to rebuild your product every time you wanted to incorporate a new data type, things are going to move really slowly—as slowly as innovation in the electronic health records space. I was going through my mother's old papers recently, and she started working on electronic health records back in the early 1970s. The broad vision that she articulates in those papers is not that different from what it looks like today, and we're still trying to achieve it. That's because these systems aren't built using a modular, layered open architecture.

Open mHealth is creating that modularity in the market of mobile health. We need that modularity not just in the pipes we send data through, but also at a higher level, so that different technical systems can know what exactly is coming in, and design around it.

DN: How do device and app makers see what you are doing?

DE: When you download an app, or buy a wearable device, the data you generate often goes up to a server owned by that company. By using common ways of communicating that data to and from the server, it becomes infinitely easier for others to build meaningful products on top of the data. The company won't have to do anything different with their product, but once that data is up on the server, others can come along and use that data to provide relevant medical recommendations or support clinical decision making—subject to authorization by the consumer of course. Imagine a doctor has patients with chronic pain, and those patients each come in using a different tracking app for pain. The clinician might then also want them monitor their dietary intake, for which they could use a completely different app. It's hard to gain meaningful insight from isolated apps. By having standardized data interfaces, we can create integrated experiences that work across applications, even as the specific applications change.

Currently, we are in the bootstrapping stage. Companies will say things like "when you show me that everybody else is doing this, I'll jump on it too." To move things forward, we are developing additional components, like connectors and end-user facing products, so that companies can gain utility more immediately.

DN: What does "open" mean in Open mHealth? Open data?

DE: No. There are three ways that "open" is commonly used, and they get confused frequently. "Open source" means that the computer code is readable and changeable. Most software is based on some open source code—those are the things that you don't want to rebuild all the time, and open source lets you build faster by reusing components. Open source is great for common components, and then you can layer proprietary pieces of code on top—what a company would consider its "secret sauce." For example, our reference data storage unit, which helps people to pull in, store, and process data from different sources, is completely open source.

The second "open" is "open data." That has to do with opening data, such as from governments, and making datasets more publicly available. Researchers want to be able to get to data that originates in larger agencies and companies. To enable this, institutions usually try to sanitize their datasets. They have to make sure they include data only from people who opted in, and/or are aggregated to a level that cannot be associated with an individual. If you aggregate to all the women in Dawn's age bracket in Portland, you could not target an advertisement to Dawn. But if you overlay with another dataset—female social scientists who work at Intel in Portland—then there is the ability to de-identify the data. When medical researchers decline to share their data with other researchers, it's not because they are being proprietary about it, it's often because of deanonymization issues. People can use Open mHealth to generate open datasets, but that's orthogonal to what we do.

The third "open" is "open architecture," which is what we focus on. This means you have well-defined, common interfaces between different elements of your system, to enable scalable modularity, like the Internet example I gave earlier. In our case, the open architecture uses a set of data schemas which provide guidelines for formatting and describing data. Anyone can use them. Proprietary platforms like Facebook are not open platforms, but they have developed open APIs—server-level connections to Facebook—so that third parties can develop apps that connect to Facebook. Facebook is not an open architecture.

**DN:** It is interesting that when you have a developer account with Facebook, you contractually agree to not build something that competes with Facebook. They'll cut you off if you do.

**DE:** When people build to a third-party API, that's the only platform those third parties can work with. But with an open architecture, it's not just that the platform can accept many third party applications, it's also that a third party application can work over multiple platforms, without having to build a custom interface for each. It opens up the market and accelerates innovation. In the context of mobile health, there are so many different components, and not one dominant provider. Apple, Samsung, and Google have all made moves, but at least for now, there's still not just one player. Our health is a distributed, multifaceted thing.

**DN:** So what does it actually mean to have standardized ways to represent data? It sounds like you are talking about something more involved than file formats—like if I have a .json or .csv file I can email it to you and your computer can open it.

**DE:** JSON just means that the computer can read the bytes, but it doesn't know how to then make sense out of it at a semantic level. You need something beyond the JSON level—a standardized schema for a particular data type.

**DN:** I'm confused about what you mean by "schema" here.

**DE:** When you put data in an Excel spreadsheet, you define what the columns and the rows are. And you define what certain formulas are based on those columns and rows. The definition of columns and rows are your schema, and that helps software know what is contained where in the file. Open mHealth has a registry where people can publish a schema, which says "this is how you interpret data from my device or app." Then people can write software code that interprets what is encoded in the JSON in order to include it in visualizations, process it, etc. Open mHealth designs schemas to ensure the data contains all the information necessary to be usable and useful in a clinical setting. Where possible we align these schemas with existing clinical libraries, but we can't just standardize them all and then move forward because we are generating new data types all the time. It's not just HG1C [a common way to measure blood glucose levels], or body temperature, it's things like the cadence of when you are walking for ten minutes, stress signatures in your voice patterns, etc.

These are evolving, and so we need to let people define schemas[2] for representing these new, different types of data.

**DN**: Taylor's chapter [11, this volume] suggests that the data types that are emerging are pretty conservative. They reflect how we already think about what to measure (a heart rate, an episode of cycling, etc.). There's some evolution, as you say, but not a lot of innovation happening.

**DE**: He may want new kinds of data, but whatever kind of data he (or we as a society) would want is going to need to have some definition to it. A system that is going to do something with it is still going to have to know what the structure is in order to visualize it for him. So that issue is not that connected to what we're talking about here.

**DN**: I see your point, though one consequence of what he's saying is that these assumptions about data shape how it is organized. The location data ends up in one database, the heart rate another.

**DE**: Yes, but that's just dumb. When things are associated with an individual, and they all have time stamps on them, that's the kind of thing open architectures help with. It helps tie together your time series of heart rate with your time series of location.

**DN**: What does a description of data look like in Open mHealth?

**DE**: It's mostly about defining the fields of data so software knows how to parse it. Low-level data could be giving estimated latitude/longitude coordinates. Each of those is a number, associated with a time stamp, and the time zone it came from (or however you are handling time zones). You might also want to know where this data originated from. Is the blood glucose a fasting blood glucose or measured just after a meal? The fact that the values are numeric and not text, the time zone handling, the device, are all part of the "description."

Applications usually want to work at a higher level, however. An app might map one person's location as "home" and the other as "workplace." You could then have data that represents average number of hours at home per day, or the time the person left the house in the morning, or even the variance in the time a person left the house in the morning. With somebody with rheumatoid arthritis you might be looking for a behavioral biomarker to determine whether there is variability in when they leave the house in the morning, or a sudden decline. So now you are not just dealing with GPS, but encoding information at this higher level, which is around a new parameter you have just defined—a biomarker. All of those things are numbers and tags that get encoded in some way, which applications need to know in order to take an action, or visualize it.

DN: I think we in the social sciences often underappreciate just how many components there are to even the simplest dataset. How heterogeneous is this space right now? Are there commonly used levels of aggregation for example—days for stress but minute by minute for something else?

DE: It depends on what you are measuring. Whether you aggregate across a day or a week depends on what action you are informing—are you updating your medication for when you go in to the clinician once every six months, and just need a general picture of how you have been, or are you trying to figure out why something went wrong in this past week? So much depends on the purpose, and right now the space is so primitive we can't make generalizations.

DN: Perhaps if it is that use-case dependent, then the level of heterogeneity could remain fairly high. People will always want to do different things with data.

DE: I would hope so.

DN: What would an app developer have to do to get their data into Open mHealth?

DE: There are two things they have to do. First, if they want to make their app integratable with other apps, they need to implement an Open mHealth API on their server, which doesn't mean it will be automatically readable by anyone and everyone—there are permissions and authentications and so forth that app users still control. Those other apps can then do processing or visualization of that data. Second, if they are producing a new type of data that hasn't been defined yet, they need to define the schema associated with their data and publish that as part of the API so that people can appropriately make sense of it. We give support for both of those things.

DN: What would health providers, public health researchers, technology developers, etc., like to do with the level of interoperability that Open mHealth provides?

DE: The most productive path is for people to think about what they know about a condition, what they know about patients and clinicians, and then say, ideally, "This is what we want to be able observe more frequently in the course of everyday life," or "This is what we would like to help patients to do more consistently." Then we can move to [figure out] how to get proxies for that measurement, or figure out when you would want to intervene.

**DN:** It seems to me that today the discussion goes the other way—there's a notion of "there's all this new data out there, what can we make of it?"

**DE:** I'm personally not interested in looking at everything we can do [technically] and then trying to make sense of it. That's too broad, not as informed as it could be by people like Ida [Sim, clinician and other cofounder of Open mHealth] who can tell you something about the clinical context. I don't just mean doctors, but also very knowledgeable patients who understand what it is to live with that condition, and what makes a difference to them. Still, you have to do it in some systematic way. You really want the top-down [approach], but informed by the bottom-up—a co-innovation process. It's important to not just freeform this. Our collaborative tracking tool Linq,[3] for example, aims to provide a way of collecting and using data for answering specific clinical questions in a clinical setting. It is based on our understanding of what is useful in the context of clinical practice.

**DN:** We have a tendency to think that "the data" is always some low-level data—like step counts, and the problem is what you can infer from it, for better or worse. But this way of thinking doesn't put you in the more powerful position of saying we can in fact *design* the data, and make meaningful decisions about what we are actually looking for.

**DE:** Right now everyone is reacting to a particular set of artifacts at a particular time. In some senses, pedometers have been around forever—they have as much evidence as anything. It's not that step counting is meaningless, it's that mobile health is about *doing* something with data that has to inform action by the patient, the clinician, the researcher. We should be looking at those higher-level actions, and not get stuck in what we have today.

## Notes

1. www.openmhealth.org.

2. See http://www.openmhealth.org/documentation/#/schema-docs/overview for further information on how schemas work (accessed August 17, 2015).

3. www.linqhealth.co.

# 10

# Field Notes in Contamination Studies

Marc Böhlen

This text discusses two field studies in the use of biosensing technologies to detect and respond to contaminated public water sources. The first field study examined recreational waters at public beaches in Western New York, United States. The second field study examined biological contamination of essential drinking water in Yogyakarta, Indonesia. At the time this research began—in 2010—environmental biosensing was largely a topic of technical research and development in university and private sector labs, with few commercially available products. What happens when those technologies make their first steps out into the world? I will attempt to trace "live" aspects of the socio-technical development of a particular biosensing technology and show how it eventually solved long-standing biocontamination detection problems, how it introduced new ones, and how old habits and administrative inertia opposed the potential effectiveness of the system while new habits emerged.

Showing how the projects unfolded necessarily requires an attention to the materials used. I hope to show, however, that these are no mere "details" and important for the construction of information flows. Some parts of those information flows are not always reconcilable with one another, nor are they fully anticipatable, but with careful attention to both the local conditions, and technical feasibility, rounds of iteration can indeed result in a mutually beneficial, workable, though fragile, technical system.

## Calamity

Walkerton is a small town in southern Ontario, situated along the banks of the Saugeen River. In May of 2000 this unassuming town became a household name due to a cascade of events that led to the contamination of the municipal water supply. Fueled by two days of heavy rains, surface water runoff overwhelmed the ability of the ground soil to absorb the water masses. Torrential rains washed bacteria from cattle farm[1] manure into the caption area of a water well connected to Walkerton's municipal water system. This shallow well, set in highly fractured bedrock covered with only a thin layer of soil (O'Connor 2002) was neither receiving the required levels of chlorination nor being monitored according to protocol. Add to this combination of events a lack of oversight, inadequate expertise,[2] severe cuts in staffing, privatization of municipal water testing, and communication blockages,[3] and you have, with a delay expected for the incubation period of this E. coli strain,[4] the worst municipal drinking water disaster in Canadian history (Salvadori et al. 2009). At least seven people died and over 2,300 residents fell ill (Bruce-Grey Owen Sound Health Unit 2000).

## Reading Water

Prevailing water-quality diagnostic logic associates the quality of drinking water with the concentration of coliforms present in water (Fricker and Eldred 2009). Coliforms are a group of related bacteria species. In the past, the term "coliform" included all lactose-fermenting species of the family *Enterobacteriaceae*, and these are usually found in mammalian (including human) feces. From the perspective of drinking water evaluation, E. coli are important both because certain strains can be dangerous in and of themselves, as the Walkerton cased illustrated, and because they are indicators, or cofactors, whose presence indicates the presence of other hard-to-detect bacteria that are in turn very harmful to human beings (Quilliam et al. 2011). Additionally, and important for the diagnostic logic, E. coli are absent when other harmful bacteria are absent in water.

In the wake of the Walkerton public calamity, a novel optical bacterial detection technology was developed by a group of scientists led by Stephen Brown (n.d.) and the departments of Chemistry, Environmental Studies, and Microbiology and Immunology at Queen's University in Kingston, Ontario. The team's technical approach was based on advances in laser technology applied to environmental problems in the 1990s (Panne and Niessner 1997) and luminescence spectroscopy (Aaron 2000; Gauglitz 2005). This research contributed directly to understanding that fluorescence from bacterial interaction with a growth medium (created by compounds that absorb ultraviolet light and emit visible light) can be generated at the sensitivity level required to detect bacteria in aqueous solutions in minute concentrations. More challenging was developing enzymes that could be used as catalysts for specific bacterial conditions, as well as designing sample equipment to enable the enzyme to be immobilized onto an appropriate interface to an optical fiber. Creating growth media and handling procedures was laborious, but optimized through trial and error, with modifications throughout early product release.

So how, then, can fluorescence be used to detect E. coli, and why does this matter? The EB16 (Endetec B-16) used in our field studies is a laboratory-grade bacterial detection system built upon the fluorescence mechanism I described. The EB16 can in principle be used to process a wide array of biological agents. The commercially available desktop system can process up to sixteen samples simultaneously and detect coliforms with single-cell sensitivity. While these are major improvements in and of themselves, the device substantially reduces the amount of time required to detect bacteria. Some details might be helpful. The composition of the reaction media together with the laser wavelength defines the system's ability to detect a particular biological target. A test run begins when a cartridge with the growth medium and the water sample is inserted into the instrument, allowing coliform bacteria to multiply in a temperature-controlled environment. The system can determine in real time the levels of bacteria growth (in colony forming units, CFUs). As the bacteria begin to multiply, they emit enzymes[5] that interact with the growth medium and generate detectable fluorescent molecules. The level of this fluorescence is gaged by its effect on an ultraviolet light source that is reflected from a film at the bottom of the test media bottle.[6] When a light detector detects that the luminescence signal has crossed a particular strength threshold, the device registers a "bacteria present" event.

The time between the start of the test and the registration of the bacteria present event is the time to detect (TTD). The TTD value is indicative of the total bacteria concentration, with higher concentrations resulting in lower TTDs. Similarly, the lower the concentration of bacteria, the longer the test process must continue, which results in higher TTDs. Highly contaminated samples can be evaluated within a few hours, and lightly contaminated samples in the single cell level will take up to sixteen hours to evaluate. Since the bacteria growth is exponential in time, a logarithmic plot of CFU vs. TTD is linear and can be used as a calibration function (Brown 2012). This is important as the TTD is an operational parameter and only meaningful for water quality if it can be mapped to an existing and established metric such as CFU. While the CFU world operates as a spatial practice of visual detection and tallying, the TTD world is temporal. It is the believable and reconstructible mapping from

TTD to CFU that allows this new class of biosensing system to establish itself as part of mainstream water-quality measurement practice. This temporal regime has furthermore implications for the system's efficiency, and consequently its ability to disrupt existing biocontamination evaluation frameworks that operate across days, not hours. The case studies that follow illustrate these dynamics.

Finally, this particular design enables laypeople without formal lab training to perform drinking water–quality assessments. As opposed to established and widely deployed methods such as membrane filtration and the most probable numbers approach, no visual interpretation is required, removing human expertise but also human error from the evaluation loop. As such, this biosensor system is part of a new wave of "convenient" non-expert devices that are bringing previously cost-prohibitive biosensing technologies to locations and situations that large-scale laboratories could never reach.[7]

## Swimming Pleasures

Before I dive into two biotechnology field studies I would like to add a few comments on my research practice. I am neither an anthropologist nor a scientist, but an artist-engineer.[8] As such, I employ a cross-disciplinary medley of methods from handicrafts, robotic hardware and software design, studio-garage practice, as well as critical science studies. In my engineering/art practice, often I am looking to surface technical and material challenges and bring them into real-life existence. This methodological mix is highly useful to create technical systems that work both technically and socially, but it does not yield an overarching theory of biosensors' impact on the world.

The first field study addressed the challenge of assessing the quality of recreational waters in Western New York. The Glass Bottom Float (GBF) project's goal was to algorithmically identify a good day to go for a swim. In order to address this seemingly simple problem, my research team and I built a floating robot with a sensor system that included use of the EB16 alongside other sensors to detect sixteen water and weather parameters in real time. Additionally, we interviewed over 600 beach visitors in 2012 and asked them in short anonymous interviews about their perception of the water conditions. Daily measurements from the EB16 with the data from the physical sensors determined the chemical and bacterial contamination levels at the beach. Furthermore, these data were mapped to a metric of swimming quality, the Swimming Pleasure Measure, which we developed and made available to the general public (Clark et al. 2013).

In New York State where GBF was operational, public beaches are subject to bacterial contamination tests during the swimming season in weekly to daily intervals. Beach operation staff members collect water samples from a swimming area in knee-deep water with special equipment and transfer the samples to a state-certified water analysis lab in an ice box.[9] The samples are then subject to a membrane filter method test to evaluate the concentration of E. coli. Lab results are available about thirty-six hours later and faxed (a paper trail is often required) to the corresponding beach manager. If the result exceeds 235 cfu/100ml, New York State regulations require the issuance of a public health notice ("swimming advisory"), or even beach closure until further notice.[10]

One problem with this unwieldy procedure is the duration of the process. By the time the lab results are available to the beach manager, the data are outdated; water conditions change faster than the sampling regimes can generate results. During experiments at one particularly problematic Western New York Beach (Woodlawn Beach), daily laboratory test results showed positive-negative oscillations. But because these official lab results were always over a day old, the responses (beach closings) oscillated out of sync; the time lag left contaminated beaches open and clean beaches closed. The EB16, in contrast, made the transport of samples to a remote lab unnecessary. Evaluation occurred on site in a temporary office installed at the beach, producing results the same day the samples were collected,[11] undoing the diurnal delay cycle.

Our project took the approach that a "good day to swim" was both a subjective experience as well as an environmental condition detectable by sensors. This approach allowed us to determine the best relative swimming conditions during the summers we conducted our tests.[12] But to our surprise, even an array of statistical tests failed to find significant relationships between the data collected from the sensors, including the EB16, and the interview results from the beach visitors. The most salient feature for our beach visitors was the smell of the beach. Foul odor from even small amounts of decaying sea grass would "put off" visitors even when the waters were bacterially unremarkable. Likewise, on days where the waters were less ideal—as determined by the suite of sensors—but no odors were noticeable, interviewees found no fault with the beach water.[13] This massive disconnect between official beach monitoring practices and the nose of the crowd, as it were, has yet to be addressed by the environmental testing communities.

Our attempts at deploying GBF at multiple beaches generated mixed results. Several beach managers who were at first enthusiastic about the project decided not to participate in the experiments once they understood that all the collected data would be available online and to the public. Even though beach managers considered our system to be a scientific improvement, we underestimated the significance of the social organization in being able and willing to incorporate this system into its existing framework. While our results were relayed to beach management through web-enabled devices (and even direct telephone calls in one case), we made no provisions to ensure that our biosensing-supported results were used in the decision-generating process of the existing water monitoring framework. Our results appeared at inopportune times and offered evidence for unscheduled problems. Upper management maintained the existing evaluation philosophy based on increments of days, not hours, and no one knew how to change the administrative processes to accommodate the accelerated knowledge inflow. So while our system was able to change the way data was collected and managed, it was not able to change the way data was processed and acted upon.

**Airkami**

As opposed to GBF's focus on recreational waters, the Airkami project (www.airkami.org) focused on essential drinking water. Airkami (Bahasa Indonesia for "our water"), set in the Terban district of Yogyakarta, Indonesia, monitored private and public drinking water sources with the goal of finding water contamination hot spots, but also establishing administrative and technical procedures by which the observations could become effective for local residents. We began our inquiry with a survey of water wells in the Terban district. Over the course of seven months we monitored fourteen water sites: thirteen water wells and the Code River that runs from north to south through Yogyakarta.

Environmental monitoring has a patchy track record in Indonesia.[14] Government efforts in collecting and processing environmental data are notoriously inadequate. Some of the public water wells in the Terban district are tested periodically, but so infrequently as to be of no analytic use. Furthermore, the Terban residents are not informed of the results, nor are actions taken to ameliorate the dire situation that the measurements more often than not describe.

Puskesmas (Bahasa Indonesia: *Pusat Kesehatan Masyarakat*) are government-mandated community health clinics overseen by the Indonesian

Ministry of Health. The Puskesmas network serves as the government's direct contact with the population for its health care needs. Thanks to the efforts of the local project coordinator, Ilya Maharika, we were able to set up a biosensing-based well water evaluation system in the Puskesmas Gondokusuman in Terban, about one kilometer from downtown Yogyakarta. This Puskesmas served as our center of operations, with health care staff collecting water samples from the Terban wells and bringing them back to the Puskesmas for evaluation. The liaison with the Puskesmas gave our project an unofficial note of approval that assisted in convincing Terban residents of the project's potential usefulness while the experiment was set up.

The EB16 deployed in Yogyakarta was a substantially improved system. First, the device's firmware was upgraded with an improved measurement algorithm including an internal lookup table that made a calibration process unnecessary. Second, the EB16's improved measurement algorithm was coupled with a new growth medium formula, reducing both the time required to prepare the water samples as well as the time required to detect a contamination event. Earlier growth media were packaged in pellet form, requiring vigorous and time-consuming (manual) mixing. The new growth medium was produced in powder form, reducing the mixing process to a quick two-minute event. However, this improvement also made the growth media much more susceptible to the extreme levels of humidity typical of Yogyakarta's climate, resulting in spoiled test media and invalid test results. We found ourselves forced to store the growth media containers in a refrigerator, the only such device in the Puskesmas. Third, the price for each test run (effectively the price of a plastic bottle with the growth medium) had fallen from $12/test to about $5/test, making the new system an economically viable alternative to the government-staffed cumbersome laboratory tests, especially since our custom-designed IT system moved the test results from the Puskesmas to a local server, and from there to a cloud service provider for analysis and sharing.

While the calibration procedure was no longer a technical necessity, we found a new use for the calibration effort. Once our experiments were underway, local health care officials began to voice concerns about our work and demanded we procure a "water test permit." Only then did we understand how closely our experiments were being observed. At a loss, we performed a series of split sample cross-calibration tests with the local government laboratory to compare results. This exchange created a rapport with the local agency and its members, and introduced them to our "invasive" system in a social calibration process that made the permit requirement disappear in short order.

During the seven-month test period, our team was able to collect and evaluate over two hundred water samples, approximately two tests per month for each site. In general, the drinking water sources in Terban are contaminated with fecal bacteria despite state-mandated limit of zero coliform content for public drinking sources. There are strong variations among the wells, and there are strong variations across the dry and wet seasons. Since we also installed a weather monitoring system we were able to correlate weather conditions with contamination events. Our data showed statistical evidence suggesting that the water wells fall into two basic categories: those that show increased E. coli levels during the heavy rains in the wet season and those that show increased E. coli levels during the dry season. These observations were the first biosensor-supported contributions to a deeper understanding of the well-water contamination dynamics of the Terban district of Yogyakarta (Maharika et al. 2014).

Making the test results available to the general public was an important design goal of the Airkami project. We kept a running tally of the newest results online, available to the public through a web interface.[15] Usually such datasets are kept under lock, and only government officials have access to the data in Indonesia. The second vector of public notification was a messaging system that delivered a summary of all tests completed overnight by the bio-incubator system, together with a water use recommendation, to local health care providers via email. The overnight processing became a viable option largely due to the shorter test cycles achieved by the combined software and growth media updates described earlier. But not all our plans worked smoothly, making ad hoc operational adjustments necessary, and also allowing us to reflect upon some of our initial assumptions. The first approach that included sending the test results directly to Terban residents via SMS was abandoned. First, it became impractical to keep track of all the residents' mobile phone numbers as these contact numbers changed frequently and haphazardly, often in direct response to temporary offers by telecom service providers luring them into new contracts. Second, it became clear that we needed to retain human experts in the notification loop. Keeping the health care providers of the Puskesmas as trusted linkages allowed us to make sure that the detailed knowledge such as family history shared between Puskesmas and Terban residents remained a part of process.[16] Despite the improvisations, this procedure constitutes a new approach to environmental data dissemination in the Terban district of Yogyakarta.

While the EB16 does not require laboratory training to operate, it is dependent on careful and diligent sample handling. We trained over a dozen Puskesmas staff and university students to use and service the system. These efforts were offset to some degree by a staff rotation rule that requires staff to move from one Puskesmas to another every two years. Without a doubt, the new system did increase the work and cognitive load for staff. Since our system was not part of the required task set, these extra efforts generated some friction among staff members dealing with water sample collection. The test automation reduces the number of required laboratory staff, but in turn necessitates the training of more flexible, "general purpose" health-care professionals. The combination of IT networking, data management, and sample preparation requires a type of health-care worker comfortable working across knowledge domains, and this new type of professional is not available at the Puskesmas level. It has also become clear that an additional effort in critically evaluating the results and the apparatus that generates the data needs to be put in place. In Indonesia, water-quality evaluation is the domain of the laboratory technicians, but their "replacement" by the networked bio-incubator generates the potential for a disconnect between laboratory work and health care delivery. A further side effect is the friction introduced by the waste disposal. The recommended procedure of diluting processed media fluids with 10 percent bleach and then adding the mix to the waste water system assumes that the cocktail flows into a much larger waste water network.[17] Similarly the manufacturer's declaration of used sample test bottles as "medical waste" implies the existence of a robust medical waste processing system, which is hardly the case in Indonesia or other emerging economies.

The new biosensing system is effective at detecting bacterial contamination, and the notification network does allow the knowledge to be shared as never before. But there was still a missing link, a missing connection between the sensors, computers, and people. We needed to add a way to enable the Terban residents to be more than recipients of data produced by fancy technologies. We needed a link between the new knowledge produced by the biosensing system and the existing daily habits of Terban residents. Our first attempt at this only got us so far.

In Javanese, *kemrengseng* describes the onset of the "rolling boil," a concept the Terban residents intuitively understand. A large majority of waterborne bacteria die when exposed to temperatures above 100°C (Sodha et al. 2011), and so boiling beyond *kemrengseng* is a practical and effective disinfectant. Our tests showed that even highly contaminated water samples collected from the Code River were E. coli and total coliform free after at least one minute of exposure to a rolling boil after *kemrengseng*. The ability to detect the *kemrengseng* moment without the aid of technical equipment is the key to creating a viable contextual response to the biosensor knowledge, and so we integrated the *kemrengseng* moment into a water treatment recommendation algorithm that evaluates the results from the biosensing system. This simple algorithm checks the newest lab results (E. coli and total coliforms) and suggests the use of the established water boiling practice to achieve *kemrengseng* and maintain this state for at least one minute on water taken from any well with E. coli levels greater than zero. Early evidence had suggested that some wells were drinkable at least some of the time, which would have made notification helpful. In practice, we found such extensive contamination that the need for *kemrengseng* was constant, which reduced the usefulness of notification.

In the recreational beach water experiments, our efforts culminated in the making and sharing of the multidimensional data along various vectors, including mobile media and public discussion on topics related to water quality right at the beach, during peak hours of activity. In the Terban situation, data and discussions could not be the end goal. Where clean drinking water is a luxury, a water monitoring system that only generates more data (and more bad news) is simply not good enough.

## Banking with Water

In Yogyakarta, the lack of effective governmental control of many aspects of everyday life works to the advantage of bottom-up initiatives. Indeed, daily life in Indonesia is full of "double systems"; local efforts addressing specific unmet needs in short time frames versus large-scale bureaucratic government initiatives lumbering along. At times these efforts complement each other but often the opposite is the case. The fact that there are usually two ways to get things done in Indonesia can be a potent experiment enabler. In architecture and urban planning communities, the culture of "informality" has been discussed in the context of its potential to deliver urban revitalization and community engagement in various forms (McFarlane 2012; Balducci et al. 2011; Dovey and Rajarho 2009). Likewise, the concept of distributed water care infrastructure with community-level engagement has been discussed among water resource management professionals (Makropoulos and Butler 2010; Henriques and Louis 2001). Finally, the original scope of the research agenda that supported Airkami and GBF did not include public and urban-scale consequences of biosensing. The project was predefined as a sensing project; it did not allow for adequate handling of the problems that sensors identified, but were unable to solve. All these factors played a role in the making of the subsequent project, WaterBank.

Stung by the GBF experiment's inability to directly influence actionable responses to the new biosensor insights, we decided to make use of the informal structures particular to the Indonesian condition in order to ensure that the insights into contamination dynamics we acquired through the new sensing system (as well as people's responses to it) could be integrated into daily water consumption habits. Not only did the sensing system allow us to find dynamics between rainfall and well water quality, but it also served as a "boundary process" through which we could "detect" existing water care practices. One interesting aspect of the Indonesian informality is the division of health care into two related but distinct realms. The first one is organized by the Ministry of Health as a top-down centralized and national apparatus. The Puskesmas network, into which the monitoring system Airkami is integrated, is the lowest branch of this system and reaches out to the general population for general health care needs. The second realm is a bottom-up system integrated into the RW (*Rukun Warga*, "harmonious citizens"). The network of RWs is in turn divided into RTs, *Rukun Tetangga* ("harmonious neighborhood"). The RWs organize the administration of day-to-day neighborhood affairs, including local building permits, land use disputes and water well access, for example. The decision mechanisms within the RW are the responsibility of local residents and their representatives. In practice, an RW with 70 and more families operates autonomously with voluntary services provided by the community members and decides most matters of significance to the local residents without government interference. As such, the RW builds and maintains the social glue typical of the *kampung* ("village") society. Once we had devised the plan to create WaterBank, the local PI Ilya Maharika built a working relationship with the head of the Terban RW, Pak Ulun. By placing WaterBank into the RW network, we enabled Terban residents, as opposed to government officials, to be in charge of the project.

WaterBank is a water filter and water distribution network. WaterBank processes water from a *Belik Ayu* ("beautiful spring"[18]) through a multistage filter system. The first filter step removes solids such as sand, slime, and rust. The next steps pass the water through a reverse osmosis system, a two-stage ultraviolet filter and ozone infusion to neutralize any remaining bacteria. This clean water is then crafted into remineralized water through a post-filter containing basalt from Mount Merapi and gneiss, feldspar, and quartz from the mountains surrounding the Glacier du Mont Miné in Switzerland. This post-filter system is based on previous research performed for the related "WaterBar" project.[19] As a result, Terban residents have the cleanest, freshest, and fanciest water in the vicinity. WaterBank is made meaningful by performing more than only useful cleaning operations, purposely defying groupthink of emerging markets experts suggesting "no frills products" for the poor (Karamchamdi, Kubzansky, and Frandano 2009). For example, every time someone fills a canister of water at the WaterBank, a small portion is redirected to the adjacent fish pond. This "wasted" water is a visible and audible reminder of the efforts required to create the valuable resource and an investment in the health of the fish that eventually land on Terban residents' dinner plate.

WaterBank can produce up to 400 liters of filtered water per day, and its output is part of the ongoing water-monitoring regime. A group of Terban residents, the PKK (*Pembinaan Kesejahteraan Keluarga*), who manage community resources and conflicts within the RW, have taken charge of the day-to-day operation of WaterBank. They have set the cost of one canister (nineteen liters) of WaterBank water at 4,000 rupiah, about $0.4. The water is free of fecal contamination and considered by Terban inhabitants to be very tasty. About ten canisters of WaterBank water are sold daily as of this writing, and proceeds from sales now cover the cost of electricity and filter replacements. WaterBank has regular customers, and a new snack shop, hoping to make use of WaterBank water for specialty drinks, has sprung up a few doors down the road. WaterBank is a new kind of biosensing-enabled water culture, uniquely enabled by the affordances and challenges of life in Yogyakarta.

However, the future of Airkami and WaterBank remain uncertain. The Ministry of Health has yet to decide on how to make use of the biosensing prototype system. At the time of this writing, it seems possible that Airkami might become a model for integrating a new private effort into the public health care system by, for example, offering premium water test services (as demonstrated by our system) to private clients. While such private-public partnerships promise to improve inefficient public services, there is increasingly conclusive evidence that entrepreneurs tend to favor servicing well-heeled customers at the cost of servicing the poor (Gero et al. 2013; Graham and Marvin 2001). It seems possible, and likely, that the diligent monitoring of the public wells currently in place will suffer through this revenue generation-focused service model.

It is too early to evaluate whether Airkami and WaterBank will indeed have a lasting impact on water care efforts in Terban. Not only is the biosensing system's operational framework still unstable, but also a culture of effective responses to this new class of data, beyond our limited intervention, has yet to establish itself. Possibly the most effective avenue of pursuing this next level of engagement might come from the extended urban planning community's attempts to build bridges between ad hocisms ingrained in the informalities of everyday Indonesian *kampung* life and long-term but grassroots-cognizant urban planning efforts aimed at organizing responses to rapid urban expansion (Porter et al. 2011).

The role of data repositories and IT management is interesting in this regard. Might one consider data in remote networks scattered across the globe the appropriate form of sharing information and enabling collaborative efforts in managing *kampung* data, or is a nonlocal backup plan simply yet another form of colonial control in disguise? The efficiencies generated through the remote computing elements within Airkami (Maharika et al. 2014) give the project data processing robustness that local-provider exclusive solutions cannot obtain. Yet these conveniences come at the cost of new dependencies on systems operating in other countries, and on data transmission networks under foreign control. New approaches to making global IT systems "work" for emerging economies are of essence. Certainly more than general positions (Irani et al. 2010) are required to design effective and empowering solutions.

## Biosensing and the Technological Imaginary

I have traced the "live" socio-technical trajectories as I worked with them, operating close to the materials and attending to the social relationships. By doing both at the same time, the complex interdependencies of the social, cultural, institutional, and material came to the fore. In many ways, they defy tidy summing up. Having done this concrete design work in ways that responded to the social relations involved, I offer some final thoughts on biosensing not as a technology, but as a conduit for aspirations.

Indonesia's foray into network technology (Barker 2014) and its uniquely identity-focused approach to the deployment of satellite technology have been described (Barker 2005) as examples of a new technological imaginary (Griffin 2002) particular to the national cultural sensitivities of Indonesia. I find the concept of the Indonesian technological imaginary a useful mechanism by which to explain the keen interest in state-of-the-art biosensing system in Yogyakarta.[20] This new technology is sensitive enough to robustly and cheaply detect coliform bacteria in the single colony concentration, levels which Indonesian immune systems likely have become accustomed to.[21] As such this system detects much more than anyone in Indonesia needs to know, with potentially embarrassing consequences.[22] I interpret the keen interest in this class of technology, despite its potential for embarrassment, as a desire to be accepted as a respected player within the global environmental monitoring community. All too often Indonesia is associated with rampant environmental degradation, and its antiquated slash and burn practice to clear large swaths of tropical forest for lucrative palm oil plantations, which regularly generates smog for, and ridicule and rage from its more developed neighbors.[23] As such, biosensing might operate as a technological imaginary as well as a technological trampoline that allows Indonesia to temporarily demonstrate capabilities[24] only its better-off neighbors have been able to develop or integrate into the urban infrastructure.

## What Spreads? Biosensing the Public Realm

Biosensing as a technological imaginary is not restricted to the Indonesian situation. Biosensing also provides an opportunity to "review" the very objects it applies itself to. Consider the convenience with which contamination events can now be tracked and traced, and how biosensing produces new artifacts. Consider the category of total coliforms the EB16 (and other similar biosensing systems) so precisely can tally. As in established laboratory procedures, the new biosensing system builds the "totalizing category" operationally,[25] meaning the category is defined by the particular method used to evaluate the category. But total coliforms include coliform strains found in soils, plants, and grains; they can literally be found almost everywhere. This catch-all condition artificially elevates what is operationally detectable to imagined health risks: and this potential imagination is encouraged by the ease with which these measurements can now be made, diminishing the incentive to question the categorization.

Biosensing shared resources makes explicit "what is lived with," what we share voluntarily and involuntarily. As our experiments reconfirm, there are more than biological questions at stake, and a return, if only temporarily, to earlier contagion studies (Goffey 2005), (Thaker 2005) might be helpful. The nonbiological dimensions of biomedia and contamination have been recognized as significant by several authors in the past. The metaphorical (Serres 1982 [1980]), affective (Brennan 2004) and political (Sampson 2011) dimensions of contamination have been discussed. Our experiments suggest an additional dimension, enabled by new technologies, spanned by the quotidian making of measurements: tracing contamination, once the measurement process becomes easy, convenient, and subject to administrative logic. Importantly, this new convenience belies the ill-defined effort required to follow the chains of contamination across technical and administrative barriers, from animals and human beings through invisible water pathways back to human beings and shared places and shared experiences, exposing what is involuntarily connected but temporarily separated.

Consider the consequences of a (speculative) biosensing system that could detect airborne bacteria in real time and monitor potential outbreaks of colds and flus in public spaces. Public transportation systems of bustling global cities would be perfectly suited for such a system; a dream come true for public health care officials, until a mob of bus users decides to attack a single individual who has just been flagged by this sensing system as ill and contagious. The problem this toy idea makes evident is that "detection" calls for action; it opposes indifference. But what if there are no action plans, or what if even well-intentioned public health-care rules are unpalatable to the public?

City life depends on informal contracts as much as it does on official rules of conduct. If biosensing is to become a nondestructive force within public life, it needs to become more than a tallying operation or a warning system. The "reading" of these new data requires a different kind of literacy and concern than the "reading" of weather patterns, traffic flows, or financial transactions; biosensing produces more intimate data. This uninvited intimacy requires us to connect across multiple levels the numerical and the cultural consequences of biosensing into an expanded cross-disciplinary lived calibration process with checks and balances, but also with hooks for actions to respond to the insights and embarrassments biosensing has the capacity to produce.

## Notes

1. The farm and even the cattle from which the bacteria originated were identified as part of various investigations following the catastrophe. The farmer was not found to be at fault because he "followed proper practices" (O'Connor 2002), which included the uncontrolled distribution of as much manure as cattle farm produce.

2. Key individuals (the Koebel brothers) were found to have acted with negligence and malice, entering phony data into a logbook instead of making the required (residual chlorine) measurements. However, investigators acknowledged that the brothers' actions were partly due to lacking the education and training required to understand the links between chlorination, E. coli contamination, and health risk.

3. One of the factors that prevented a rapid response was a lack of expecting the unusual. The symptoms reported were consistent with E. coli O157:H7. However, infection with E. coli O157:H7 is most commonly associated with food, not water—and referred to for this reason as "the hamburger disease" (O'Connor 2002). Also, there was no practical framework in place to spread the news among the residents of the rural community.

4. E. coli O157:H7 infection has a median incubation period of three to four days (Bruce-Grey Owen Sound Health Unit 2000).

5. Enzyme-substrate tests have now become common in optical biosensing systems. In this case the bacteria-produced enzymes β-D-galactosidase indicate the presence of total coliforms, and β-D-glucuronidase indicate E. coli (Habash and Johns 2009; Endetec B-16 n.d.).

6. The optical detection is based on byproducts of hydrolysis cleavage (splitting of a compound into fragments by addition of water) of a proprietary growth medium to which the water sample is added. Details can be found in the U.S. EPA test procedure approval document (EPA 2014).

7. The EB16 system received formal full approval from the U.S. EPA in June 2014. Regulatory approvals in other parts of the world are currently pending as well (personal email correspondence with Patrick Wolfe, Endetec, May–June 2014).

8. www.realtechsupport.org.

9. EPA water sample handling procedures are elaborately outlined in Quality Assurance Project Plan (QAPP) documents that describe every aspect of the sample collection, including custody protocols regulating the hand-off of samples between sample collectors and laboratory staff. See http://www.dec.ny.gov/docs/water_pdf/waveqapp.pdf for a 2014 New York State QAPP designed for water assessment by volunteers (accessed September 2014).

10. The process that regulates the definitions of these warnings (advisory vs. precautionary advisory or swimming restriction, for example) varies by state and even county in the United States.

11. During the experiments in 2011 and 2012, the EB16 firmware version required site-specific calibration for optimum performance in midrange contamination conditions. The calibration required the collection of a representative set of samples across the measurement spectrum, from noncontaminated to highly contaminated examples. Each of these samples was split and tested simultaneously at the state-certified lab and by the EB16 on site. Once a concordance between the baseline measurements (state lab) and the EB16 was established on the split sample set, measurements were performed only with the EB16. This calibration procedure was time consuming, costly, and impractical.

12. Other insights included, for example, the observation that winds from the east tended to increase the coliform levels for this particular beach.

13. The number of people at the beach varied considerably. A lifeguard who volunteered for an informal interview claimed to have observed a noticeable correlation between the number of people at the beach on a given day and the weather forecast as pronounced by a popular local radio host.

14. In particular, enforcement of procedures and waste water system maintenance are enduring problems (Giltner et al. 2013). Taylor for example, claims that "less than 10 per cent of the 150 sludge treatment facilities constructed in the 1990s were still functional by 2009 and ... less than 4 per cent of Indonesia's septage is treated at a treatment plant" (Giltner et al. 2013).

15. Airkami data, 2014, http://54.235.133.52/hasil_air_25.php, accessed August 31, 2015.

16. All too often the need to generate information technology–enabled efficiencies is applied indiscriminately. This is one good example of the benefits of applying the efficiencies selectively, and investing the gains at the end of the communication chain.

17. One of the health care staff was particularly concerned about the effect of the bleach mix on the bacterial flora of the health care center's small septic tank. He chose not to add the bleach, enduring the putrid odor from the used media and disposed the smelly test media directly into the septic tank.

18. Our biosensing system found the water from the Belik Ayu to be contaminated with fecal bacteria in concentrations far beyond drinkable limits, making an intervention all the more necessary.

19. http://www.vilcek.org/gallery/dartboard/marc-bohlen/index.html, accessed September 2014.

20. Our biosensing system and supporting technology were placed in the prayer room of the Puskesmas. Space constraints alone would hardly have necessitated this choice.

21. Personal communication with Dr. Riska Novriana, MD, a Puskesmas Terban physician. In particular the "total coliform" category might overestimate real risk to local immune systems. The first few experimental batches of water produced by WaterBank contained on the order of 100cfu/ml and were consumed by Terban residents with no consequences.

22. The Indonesian government officially mandates a zero E. coli concentration for all drinking water sources. New biosensing regimes might finally show the real extent of the water contamination problem, should the system become widely deployed.

23. This blog has a reference to the original media coverage of the 2013 burnings: http://ifonlysingaporeans.blogspot.ch/2013/06/pm-accepts-haze-apology-urges-swift.html, accessed August 3, 2015. For an earlier and more in-depth description of the problem, see Heather Augustyn, "A Burning Issue—Palm Oil Shows Promise as a Biofuel, But the Environmental Cost of Production Can Be High," *World Watch Magazine*, July/August 2007, Volume 20, No. 4, Worldwatch Insti-

tute, http://www.worldwatch.org/node/5136, accessed August 3, 2015.

24. National sensitivities concerning a lack of technological sophistication have become apparent on several fronts recently. In late 2013, for example, Indonesia was the "victim" of an eavesdropping operation orchestrated by Australian surveillance authorities, resulting in a full-scale diplomatic row between the two traditionally friendly nations: Rod McGuirk, "Australia Reportedly Spies on Indonesia President," *Jakarta Post*, November 18, 2013, http://www.thejakartapost.com/news/2013/11/18/australia-reportedly-spies-indonesia-president.html, accessed September 2014.

25. See http://www.standardmethods.org/, accessed September 2014. The new category of enzyme-based detection methods, including the optical biosensing approach of the EB16, makes use of the fact that approximately 98 percent of the Escherichia group produce β-D-glucuronidase, making this method more sensitive (Fricker and Eldred 2009) to the presence of coliforms, but also changing the meaning of the term "total coliforms" as additional genera now become part of the "total" category.

## References


Aaron, J. 2000. "What's New in Luminescence Spectroscopy: Applications and Recent Trends." *Analysis* 28 (8): 647–648.

Balducci, L., J. Boelens, T. Hillier, C. Nyseth, and C. Wilkinson. 2011. "Introduction: Strategic Spatial Planning in Uncertainty: Theory and Exploratory Practice." *Town Planning Review* 82 (5): 481–501.

Barker, J. 2014. "Engineers and Political Dreams: Indonesia's Internet in Cultural Perspective." http://homes.chass.utoronto.ca/~barkerj/research/technology.html. Accessed September 2014.

Barker, J. 2005. "Engineers and Political Dreams. Indonesia in the Satellite Age." *Current Anthropology* 46 (5): 703–727.

Brennan, T. 2004. *The Transmission of Affect*. Ithaca and London: Cornell University Press.

Brown, S. 2012. "Methodology for Implementing the ENDETEC TECTA B16 for Estimation of E. coli Levels." Tech Report. May 29. Kingston, Ontario: Veolia Water Solutions.

Brown, S. n.d. Website at Queens University Department of Chemistry: http://www.queensu.ca/ensc/faculty/reg-faculty/stephen-brown.html. Accessed September 2014.

Bruce-Grey Owen Sound Health Unit. 2000. Bruce-Grey Owen Sound Health Unit Waterborne Outbreak of Gastroenteritis Associated with a Contaminated Municipal Water Supply, Walkerton, Ontario, May–June 2000. *Canada Communicable Disease Report* (20): 170–173. October 15.

Clark, B., M. Böhlen, J. Dalton, J. Atkinson, D. Blersch, and L. Yang. 2013. "Another Day at the Beach: Combing Sensor Data with Human Perception and Intuition for the Monitoring and Care of Public Recreational Water Resources." In

*2013 9th International Conference on Intelligent Environments (IE)*, 37–44. July 16–17. Athens, Greece.

Dovey, K., and W. Raharjo. 2009. "Becoming Prosperous: Informal Urbanism in Yogyakarta." In *Becoming Places: Urbanism / Architecture / Identity / Power*, ed. Kim Dovey, 79–102. London and New York: Routledge.

Endetec B-16. n.d. http://www.endetec.com/endetec/ressources/files/1/20106,17140,TECTA-Brochure-EN-1.pdf. Accessed September 2014.

EPA. 2014. Expedited Approval of Alternative Test Procedures for the Analysis of Contaminants Under the Safe Drinking Water Act; Analysis and Sampling Procedures. https://www.federalregister.gov/articles/2014/06/27/C1-2014-14369/expedited-approval-of-alternative-test-procedures-for-the-analysis-of-contaminants-under-the-safe. Accessed August 2015.

Fricker, C., and B. Eldred. 2009. "Identification of Coliform Genera Recovered from Water Using Different Technologies." [December.] *Letters in Applied Microbiology* 49 (6): 685–688.

Gauglitz, G. January 2005. "Direct Optical Sensors: Principles and Selected Applications. " *Analytical and Bioanalytical Chemistry* 381 (1): 141–155.

Gero, A., N. Carrard, J. Murta, and J. Willetts. 2013. *Private and Social Enterprise Engagement in Water and Sanitation for the Poor: A Systematic Review of Current Evidence*. Sydney: Institute for Sustainable Futures, University of Technology.

Giltner, S., M. Warsono, B. Darmawan, I. Blackett, and K. Taylor. 2013. "Development of Urban Septage Management Models in Indonesia." *Waterlines* 32 (3) (July): 221–236. Practical Action Publishing.

Goffey, A. 2005. "Contagion." Editorial. *Fibreculture Journal* (4). http://four.fibreculturejournal.org/. Accessed September 2014.

Graham, S., and S. Marvin. 2001. *Splintering Urbanism: Networked Infrastructures, Technological Mobilities and the Urban Condition*. London and New York: Routledge.

Griffin, M. 2002. "Exploring the Technological Imaginary." PAJ: A Journal of Performance and Art 71 24 (2) (May): 120–123.

Habash, M., and R. Johns. 2009. "Comparison Study of Membrane Filtration Direct Count and an Automated Coliform and Escherichia coli Detection System for On-site Water Quality Testing." *Journal of Microbiological Methods* 79 (1): 128–130.

Henriques, J., and G. Louis. 2011. "A Decision Model for Selecting Sustainable Drinking Water Supply and Greywater Reuse Systems for Developing Communities with a Case Study in Cimahi, Indonesia." *Journal of Environmental Management* 92 (1): 214–222.

Irani, L., J. Vertesi, P. Dourish, K. Philip, and R. Grinter. 2010. "Postcolonial Computing: A Lens on Design and Development." In *Proceedings of the SIGCHI Conference on Human Factors in Computing Systems (CHI'10)*, 1311–1320. New York: ACM.

Karamchamdi, A., M. Kubzansky, and P. Frandano. 2009. *Emerging Markets, Emerging Models: Market-Based Solutions to the Challenges of Global Poverty*. Cambridge, MA: Monitor Group.

Maharika, I., M. Böhlen, Z. Yin, and L. Hakim. 2014. "Biosensing in the Kampung." In *2014 10th International Conference on Intelligent Environments (IE)*, 23–30. June 30–July 4. Shanghai, China.

Makropoulos, C., and D. Butler. 2010. "Distributed Water Infrastructure for Sustainable Communities." *Water Resources Management* 24: 2795–2816.

McFarlane, C. 2012. "Rethinking Informality: Politics, Crisis, and the City." *Planning Theory & Practice* 13 (1): 89–108.

O'Connor, D. 2002. "A Summary Report of the Walkerton Inquiry: The Events of May 2000 and Related Issues." Ontario Ministry of the Attorney General, Queen's Printer for Ontario.

Panne, U., and R. Niessner. 1997. "Laserverfahren in der Umweltanalytik." *Analytiker Taschenbuch* 16: 157–254.

Porter, L., M. Lombard, M. Huxley, A. Ingin, T. Islam, J. Briggs, D. Rukmana, R. Devlin, and V. Watson. 2011. "Informality, the Commons and the Paradoxes for Planning: Concepts and Debates for Informality and Planning/Self-Made Cities: Ordinary Informality?/The Reordering of a Romany Neighbourhood/The Land Formalisation Process and the Peri-Urban Zone of Dar es Salaam, Tanzania/Street Vendors and Planning in Indonesian Cities/Informal Urbanism in the USA: New Challenges for Theory and Practice/Engaging with Citizenship and Urban Struggle Through an Informality Lens." *Planning Theory & Practice* 12 (1): 115–153.

Quilliam, Richard S., A. Prysor Williams, Lisa M. Avery, Shelagh K. Malham, and Davey L. Jones. 2011. "Unearthing Human Pathogens at the Agricultural–Environment Interface: A Review of Current Methods for the Detection of Escherichia coli O157 in Freshwater Ecosystems." *Agriculture, Ecosystems & Environment* 140 (3–4) (March): 354–360.

Salvadori, M., J. Sontrop, A. Garg, L. Moist, R. Suri, and W. Clark. 2009. "Factors That Led to the Walkerton Tragedy." *Kidney International Supplement* Feb (112): 33–34.

Sampson, T. 2011. "Contagion Theory Beyond the Microbe." CTheory.net. November. Special issue: Theory Beyond Codes—In the Name of Security.

Serres, M. 1982. [1980]. *Le Parasite. Grasset / The Parasite*. Baltimore: John Hopkins University Press.

Sodha, S., M. Menon, K. Trivedi, A. Ati, M. E. Figueroa, R. Ainslie, K. Wannemuehler, and R. Quick. 2011. "Microbiologic Effectiveness of Boiling and Safe Water Storage in South Sulawesi, Indonesia." *Journal of Water Health* 9 (3) (September): 577–585.

Thaker, E. 2005. "Biophilosophy for the 21st Century." Ctheory.net. June. http://www.ctheory.net/articles.aspx?id=472. Accessed September 2014.

# 11

# Data, (Bio)Sensing, and (Other-)Worldly Stories from the Cycle Routes of London

Alex Taylor

What if we could capture more dynamic notions of form in which space is the result of tidal forces which may suddenly swirl, surge and swash in abrupt or drawn-out, pliant or emphatic, regular or irregular ways which close off or perpetuate arousal? What if they could accelerate and crest, swell and burst, surge and fade in ways which link motion and form? Territory still exists but it becomes a part of perpetually renaturalized movement and can be constantly redefined and shifted.

Nigel Thrift (2014, 6)

I want to tell a story about data and about how we might use it to reimagine the possibilities for humans and machines in the multiple worlds we co-inhabit. My story is an experimental one involving human, technological, and political bodies—of the human body, bicycles, built (techno-material) infrastructures, and the body politic, all of which weave their way through and into the streets of London. The story is one of promise, of something or somewhere else still only part formed, still open to more. Much more.

But first we must begin with what we have and where we are. Everybody has been talking about data and big data. From what we consume to how we tweet, data—we're told—cut through it all and thus has much to tell us. Where data are plentiful, or *big*, "More Isn't Just More," as a spread in *Wired* (June 2008) put it, "More Is *Different*."[1] But what is this difference, which worlds exactly might it affect, and how? As we well know, difference does do transformative work in/on worlds (Haraway 2003), but we need a better idea of what's at stake in this new "age" of data—how it is data might actually come to matter and make a difference.

Let us take biosensing as a thread feeding in to this rhetoric and a way to think through it. Biosensing introduces an imaginary of hybrids, of biology and machinic sensing entangled in new figurings of nature and technology. On the one hand, we are seeing advances in a new breed of sensors that are themselves biological. They consist of organisms that are, in a fashion, put to work in human-centric worlds to detect, measure, and signify. Most famous among these are the reengineered organisms designed to detect the presence of deadly pathogens in water. On the other hand, we see more conventional sensors being assembled to monitor bio-based systems. These are sensors intervening in everything from expansive ecological systems—ecosystems—to single discrete bodies. In both of these cases, biosensing illustrates the capacities for reimagining natures and technologies, and what divides them, or, to use Donna Haraway's phrase, refiguring "naturecultures" (1997).

Yet, in much the same way as Haraway's cyborg (or indeed her canine companions; Haraway 2003), my suggestion in what follows will be that biosensing—in and among other sensed data—is, today, being mobilized to cement the same old subject categories and is failing to achieve its potential to (re-)imagine—let alone do—difference. Pedestrian it may be, but by using the data I've found linked to London's public bike rental scheme and some data I've generated riding the bikes myself, my suggestion will be that what I call the data-everywhere paradigm accumulates, sorts, and aggregates data in ways that conform to very familiar "systems"; biology, the body, the machine, the city, value, wealth, and so on, are tightly policed categories, even when the data (may) suggest otherwise. My hope is to show, tentatively, that there are other possibilities to be found in these distributed and heterogeneous data, new relations we might discover and thus new worlds of difference we might come to perform. This, I hope, will be a way for us to begin talking about moving toward something or somewhere else—a difference in the making.

## Data, Clouds, and Computation

Before I get to this speculative experiment with London's rental bikes (and some of the stories surrounding them), let me say a little about what I see to be a pertinent relationship that can get overlooked in much of the hyperbole about sensing and biosensing. It's clear that the resurgence in sensing (that this book is, in part, a response to) is tightly bound up with data; impressive capacities to sense worldly phenomena have been built and these have in part led to the "deluge" in data that we are hearing so much about. However, as well as its production, what also undergirds data's proliferation is an infrastructure of storage, distribution, and computation. Much of this falls into yet another popular and much touted term, the "cloud."

The cloud references an information technology and storage infrastructure that distributes data across remote machines, and often across more than one machine, simultaneously. The burden of storage is shifted to high-capacity data centers, server farms, and so on, thus doing away with many of the attendant issues associated with local storage, such as data loss, restricted (location-/machine-dependent) access, finite capacity, and so on. These technological capacities are having a profound impact on how the presence of data is being felt in daily life. Most visibly we encounter an ever-growing army of people tethered to smartphones, tablets, wearables, and similarly connected devices, all relying on services hosted in the cloud. Also, many of us have felt, acutely, the very real and often vexing problems faced with the widespread distribution of data. It seems we quickly run into difficulties when we store, create, and share things remotely. The widely publicized furors over ownership rights and privacy with Facebook, Google, and Apple's iCloud offer insight into just how fraught the problems can be for both the providers and the consumers of cloud computing. More detailed and grounded research also shows that there is unease with the nascent cloud-based models of interacting with data and content. The long and short of it is, with our use of the cloud, we're often not sure where our digital stuff is anymore, how to keep track of it, and who else can see and get hold of it (Shklovski et al. 2014; Lindley et al. 2013).

Less visible, but more relevant to the points I want to develop are the capacities to aggregate, mine, and interpret these widely distributed data. These capacities are evident in products that would be unfamiliar to many like Amazon's *Elastic MapReduce* or Microsoft's *WindowsAzure*. With these products the capacity for computation on a vast scale underlies most of the services consumers and professionals take for granted in their daily dealings with data. For instance, the service that lets you digitally tag and comment on real brick-and-mortar places and geographical locations, *foursquare*, subjects the data its 55 million users produce to learning algorithms and long-term trend analysis, and this is all done using the cloud-based, computational services available from Amazon.

Although biosensors have yet to operate and be sold at any kind of significant scale, one doesn't need to look hard to find this model being used with biosensing technology. HealthPatch™ by Vital Connect Inc. uses sensors to measure heart rate, motion, and skin temperature. The company's purported claim is that "the HealthPatch biosensor is your solution to tracking your health and wellness or that of a loved one."[2] Putting to one side, for a moment, the imagined use of the technology,

HealthPatch is built to be coupled with other devices and services so that data are amassed and aggregated to infer a human body's status and specifically health. What I want to draw attention to here is that the viability of HealthPatch is heavily reliant not just on sensing data, but also on data aggregation and distribution across these devices and services, and in the cloud. Indeed, even though Vital Connect has a privacy policy[3] that assures "good faith" in protecting personally identifiable information, it leaves plenty of room for using the data its sensors collect. In its data integrity policy, for example, it explains it "processes personal information only for the purposes for which it was collected and in accordance with this Privacy Policy or any applicable service-specific privacy notice."

My suggestion is not that Vital Connect has any intention of breaching people's privacy or misusing personally identifiable information, but rather the vision for its biosensors is tightly bound up with what is done with the data. This is made slightly clearer in the promotional material from Aventyn Inc., the company providing the information systems platform for Vital Connect and its biosensors. On one of its webpages, Aventyn promotes the health-sector quality improvements and efficiencies it enables by producing "technologies to connect electronic patient-centric health information for anytime, anywhere, anyplace access." The benefits are realized because their products enable them to "aggregate, filter and route interoperable patient health and connected medical device asset information."[4] In short, their platform is dependent on underlying computational capacities for data aggregation and distribution—capacities that allow heterogeneous kinds of data to be brought together and put in relation to each other.

Placing this within a wider, critical dialogue, I find a lot of value in a point made by boyd and Crawford in which they highlight the importance relational networks play in big data: "Big Data is notable not because of its size, but because of its relationality to other data." (boyd and Crawford 2011, 1). What seems new then is not the data, per se, but the ways the relations are being figured. boyd and Crawford's point also alludes to the importance of the infrastructural substrate that underlies big data, that it is "big" because the structural qualities of computation and the Internet (and now the cloud) enable large and disparate, but still very particular, sets of data to be sorted, assembled, and reassembled (Graham 2005). In other words, the cuts made using big data are all about configuring connections and these connections are contingent on the particular kinds of networks that can be set in relation to one another using the new infrastructures of the web, the cloud, aggregation, and so on. Big data is about networks all the way down and my point is that biosensing and biosensors appear to be tightly knit into these networks. Indeed it would seem impossible (or at least less than adequate) to separate (bio)sensors from the capacities for drawing data together and the "coding technologies" (Wilson 2011) used to look for and produce intelligible relationships.

Data, and especially data under the rubric of big data, has certainly seen sizeable coverage of this data "mining" in the popular press, often with commentaries to fit the unfortunate allusions to Orwellian newspeak in the term. Yet there is little in the way of concerted research to examine what the less visible analytics and computation that enable data aggregation and distribution are doing in practice and what it in fact means (or could mean) for people. There seems something of a kneejerk out-of-sight-out-of-mind response here, where much like the infrastructures that underlay ordinary operation in built environments, we simply don't want to know or think about what goes on below or beneath (Star and Strauss 1999; Graham and Marvin 2001). The underworld that pervades ordinary life but remains invisible (most of the time) is seen as too dirty or, in the case of computation, complicated, and while it may on occasion worry many of us we seem prepared to think of it as "a necessary evil."

The questions begged are what in actual fact do these data services do, how do we come into contact with them (if we do), and what *might* we want them to do if we knew more about them and their potential? These, on the face of it, may seem purely human, even moral concerns. Again, the technology would appear to be simply the backbone to these usage questions, constituting the enabling infrastructures or platforms that people will eventually use. To understand what's at stake, such questions, though, evidently demand—at the very least—a depth of understanding in the technological capacities intrinsic to (bio)sensors, data, and the cloud. As I see it, also needed is a much better understanding of how data operates vis-à-vis the kinds of "techno social complexes" detailed by the geographer Steven Graham (2005). We have much to learn in how to think about people and social life in relation to citywide, geospatial data infrastructures, and what, in combination, they enact.

How then might we look past the grand claims, and recognize data and (bio)sensing for the differences they might enable; not as a panacea for everything from the ultimate market research tool to displacing the need for theory in science (Bowker 2014; Kitchin 2014), but as a means of difference-making through a distinctive assembly of techniques and resources.

## Boris Bikes

So, in broad terms, I want to argue that one useful way to think through data and (bio)sensing is in how, together, they offer particular cuts into and enactments of worldly phenomena. As I've said, in this chapter I want to experiment with both thinking and doing to explore our understandings along these lines. The exercise will be one of cutting through a set of bodies, spaces, data, computation, etc. to think about, one, what kinds of worlds are being materialized when things like biosensors are entangled in wider human–machine assemblies and, two, what other different worlds could possibly be imagined.

The particular cut I'd like to use to develop this line of thinking concentrates on the journeys people make through cities and how these intersect and entangle with data and computation. Broadly, the relations configured here are between people, their movements in cities, and the data generated and computed by these movements. My focus will be on London's public bike rental scheme that was launched in 2010 by the city's mayor, Boris Johnson (hence the nickname for the bikes: "Boris Bikes"), and a number of efforts that have been made to access and use the data the scheme generates.

Although these bike data arguably don't quite deserve the moniker big data, my hope is it will help to illustrate how data of a sizeable scale—both in terms of quantity and the duration over which it is being generated—must inevitably be seen in terms of relationality and worlds enacted. My aim is to explore how the data weave into particular individual and political motives, programmatic and computational contingencies, and the various ways people interface with the scheme at both an individual and urban scale. I want to examine how sensors and biosensors come to be a part of these always emerging assemblies, introducing data that enable yet further relations and cuts through the networks. I'll be especially interested in how the different data extend beyond the digital and how entangled relations transform the organization of the data, how people interface with it, what it comes to represent, and ultimately what worlds are made in these entangled processes and practices. In short, I want to see how data may be wasting potential when treated purely as a set of numbers to be computed and processed, as inhabiting an immaterial or ethereal cyberstructure, or representative of some set of stable phenomena. The promise, I'll speculate, is in seeing data as emergent, at one and the same time evolving in and performing particular material relations, and along unfolding trajectories.

**Some History**

In August 2010, when Mayor Boris Johnson launched the Barclays Cycle Hire scheme (privately sponsored by Barclays Bank), the promise was to make as much of the bike usage data available as possible. The data were presented as a resource for third-party developers, and London's overarching public transport organization, Transport for London (TfL), committed to supplying the data without competing in the consumer market itself. As a public authority, the unfettered availability of the data was also congruous with TfL's obligations under the UK's Freedom of Information Act.

Despite these pledges, all that was initially provided was a website listing the availability of the rental bikes, limiting not only the kinds of data made available but also useful access to it. It was left to developers with initiative to "scrape" these data from the site to build tools and mobile apps for users. Those that appeared ranged from relatively straightforward sites indicating the availability of bikes at the docking stations dotted around the city, to more innovative uses, identifying, for instance, the busiest stations or even predicting future bike and docking station availability.

Alongside this, a number of attempts were made to gain better access to the bike data. One particularly effective attempt was pursued by the developer and open data advocate Adrian Short. On the public announcement of the millionth Boris Bike journey and the surrounding fanfare, Short requested information on bike usage for these million trips. His correspondence with Transport for London is conveniently logged on the site *What Do They Know*, which keeps a record of all FoI (Freedom of Information) requests. The original request, dated October 8, 2010, asked for a data file including the following:

Journey ID
Bike ID
Time and date of the start of the journey
Time and date of the end of the journey
Origin docking station ID

Destination docking station ID

What the log of correspondence shows is TfL's apparent initial resistance to releasing the data, in full, and the date, January 5, 2011, when TfL eventually made a downloadable file available on what they call their "Developers' area." It also shows an eventual recognition of TfL's failure to fully comply with the FoI act by delaying the compliance to this request by forty-two working days more than the allotted twenty-working day limit, and not offering any reason for this delay.

As Short has documented on his own blog (Short 2011), however, it's his opinion that TfL remained in contravention of FoI, even when the data were made downloadable. He forcefully criticized London's transport authority for insisting people who download the data provide identifying details and in effect enter into a contractual agreement with TfL. As Short puts it: "So why was the data delayed. … The answer lies in TfL's desire to wrap the data in a complicated contract rather than make it available to me or anyone else directly and legally unencumbered. This might make sense in the context of some data and some data users but it's directly inimical to the aims and indeed the law of freedom of information. The data in TfL's developers' area isn't open data and it's not available to everyone."

Now, all this may seem far removed from (bio)sensing, people's everyday use of the Boris Bikes, and big data. However, the point I want to make is that these seemingly obtuse issues around TfL, FoI, and the access to the bike data provide one way to see the relations between the data, the use of the bikes, people's sense of and orientation to the wider bike rental scheme, and ultimately how bodies are figured in and move through a city. By following the data, we find very particular kinds of assemblies being enacted, ones knitted together by transport agencies, regulatory frameworks, data flows, and (political) ideals. The data come into being and flow through not just technological networks, but also a specific configuration of actors and agencies. Data come to matter, if you will, and are enacted through (individual, organizational and technological) bodies, and their relations to one another.

## A Figured City

Let us stand back for a moment and see what the data and entangled relations mean for the city as a body—and the body politic. What initiatives like Short's have ultimately resulted in is the release of a "Barclays Cycle

Hire availability feed" for tracking the use of individual Boris Bikes. Through direct requests as well as their innovative uses of the available data, Short and others continually pushed TfL to produce a viable system for accessing a real-time data feed of bike usage. These efforts have also mobilized at least some of the development initiatives being coordinated under an open data mandate.

For example, Short was one of the people who, early on, scraped data from TfL's bike rental scheme website, but he did so with the express intention of giving other developers better access to the data. This move to open up the data led to the release of numerous apps for visualizing bike availability, and a recognition of Short's efforts from the small development community. As a consequence, it also offered Boris Bike users an early way to locate the docking stations across the city and check availability either online using a web browser or apps developed for smartphones. The effect was thus an interleaving of the bike networks, data, and usage. Each came to be meaningful and indeed useful with respect to the other.

One striking example of this intermingling is evident in the duration of rental bike journeys. When renting a bike, the first thirty minutes is defined as "free" on the official Cycle Hire website (although this does not include the "Bike Access" charge). It's not surprising then that the data show that bike journeys on average hover around twenty minutes and that well over 90 percent of all journeys fall under the "free" thirty-minute time limit. More interesting is that developers have recognized the importance of this and in some cases have included features in their apps that predict cycle times from any given docking station to another. The net result is that an urban geography emerges through calculated and predicted time intervals and most markedly the limits of thirty-minute bicycle journeys. For bike travel, at least, London comes to be figured as a city divided up into sub-thirty-minute cycle journey segments, giving shape to its own distinctive network of nodes and connections (figure 11.1).

People's movements, mass urban transport, software, code, computation, and more intermingle to materialize city (infra)structures in the making (figure 11.1a). Real-time computed bike availability data from TfL, developers computational tools used to estimate routes and times, accessible cartographic maps plotted with docking stations and road networks, and flows of people and bikes across these networks, etch a visible spatial and temporal pattern onto and into the city. From up on high, the data-infused (infra)structures enliven flows that course, like arteries, producing a shifting patchwork of macrocosms (figure 11.1b).

A

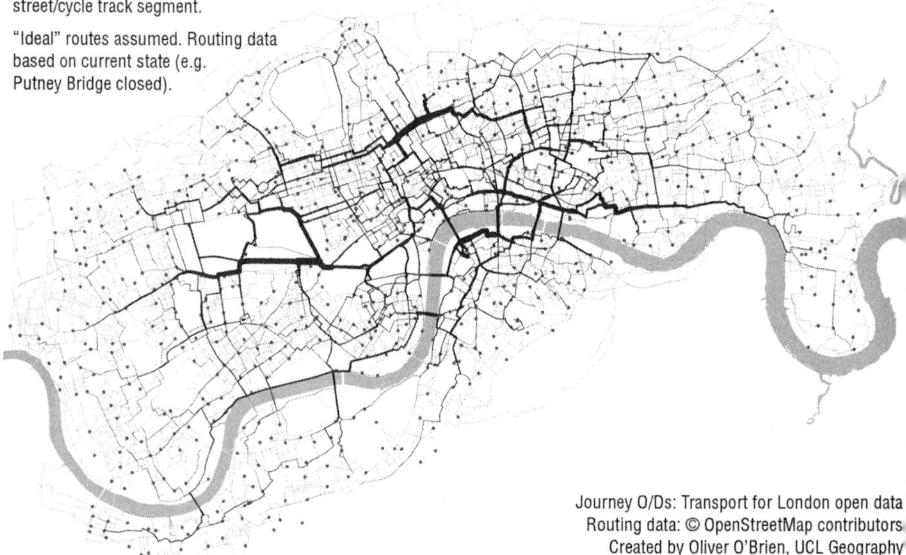


B

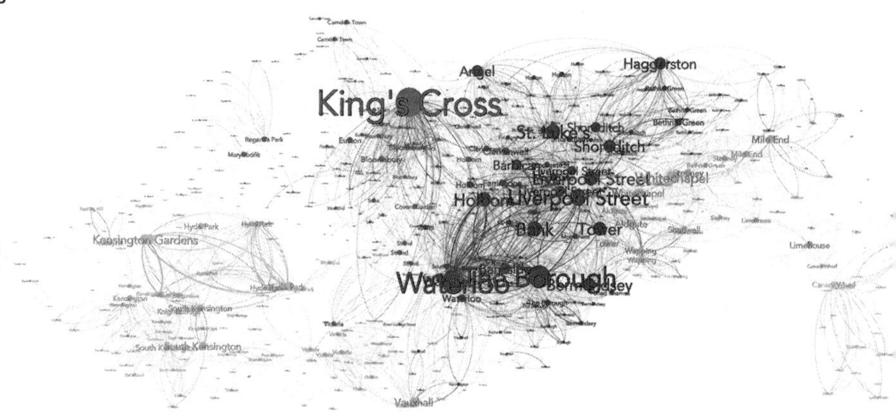


**Figure 11.1**

(a) Map of Barclays Cycle Hire usage by Oliver O'Brien (2014), showing "calculated routes" and volume of twelve million journeys between December 2013 and July 2014; and (b) "Connected clusters" of bike docking stations by James Siddle (2014).

## A Caesura

Now let us imagine things from somewhere else, from what at first glance may seem a different level of detail. To put myself in these networks of data, I have on one fine autumn day in London taken my first Boris Bike journey. My ride, on Friday, October 3, 2014, is on bike number 2175. Transport for London's publically available records show in the preceding week it being used between five to eight times a day from its starting point in a western neighborhood of London, Battersea. As I set off, the bike has rested, locked to its docking station, for almost twenty-four hours.

My journey is between two docking stations that lie at the eastern edge of the cycle scheme's cartography of routes and stops. The starting point is the Aberfeldy Street docking station, situated on a largely residential road, with rows of low-rise, rundown apartment buildings and street-fronted shops (most boarded up). Heading off, the route I take leads me further east (about five kilometers beyond the scheme's easternmost docking station), through a series of neighborhoods that, despite their proximity to the financial district, Canary Wharf, still feel a long way from London's ever-increasing prosperity and cycles of gentrification. After riding north along the popular market street of Green Street in Newham, I then head back due west to a docking station in Bow, eventually just 0.5km north of Aberfeldy Street. In total, my journey takes forty-five minutes, starting at 16:45 and ending at 17:30. The average journey time for the seventy-four rides that began at the same time, across the scheme, was fifteen minutes.

For my journey, I carry three devices that generate data. Taped to my upper chest I wear one of Vital Connect's biosensor HealthPatches (figure 11.2c), measuring my heart rate and calculating other derivatives of this including my heart rate variability (HRV).[5] To monitor activity though changes in bodily orientation and movement, I also carry a Withings Pulse 02 personal activity tracker (figure 11.2a). Finally, clipped to my coat is an Autographer (figure 11.2b), a camera device that automatically captures image sequences using, as the promotional material claims, five sensors "fused by a sophisticated algorithm to tell the camera exactly the right moments to take photos."[6] These three devices, a range of off-the-shelf biosensors or self-monitoring systems, each purport to capture in some shape or form individual physiological or bodily phenomena.

My journey—equipped with sensors—is an intentional move to the edges of London's bike rental docking stations and the associated data

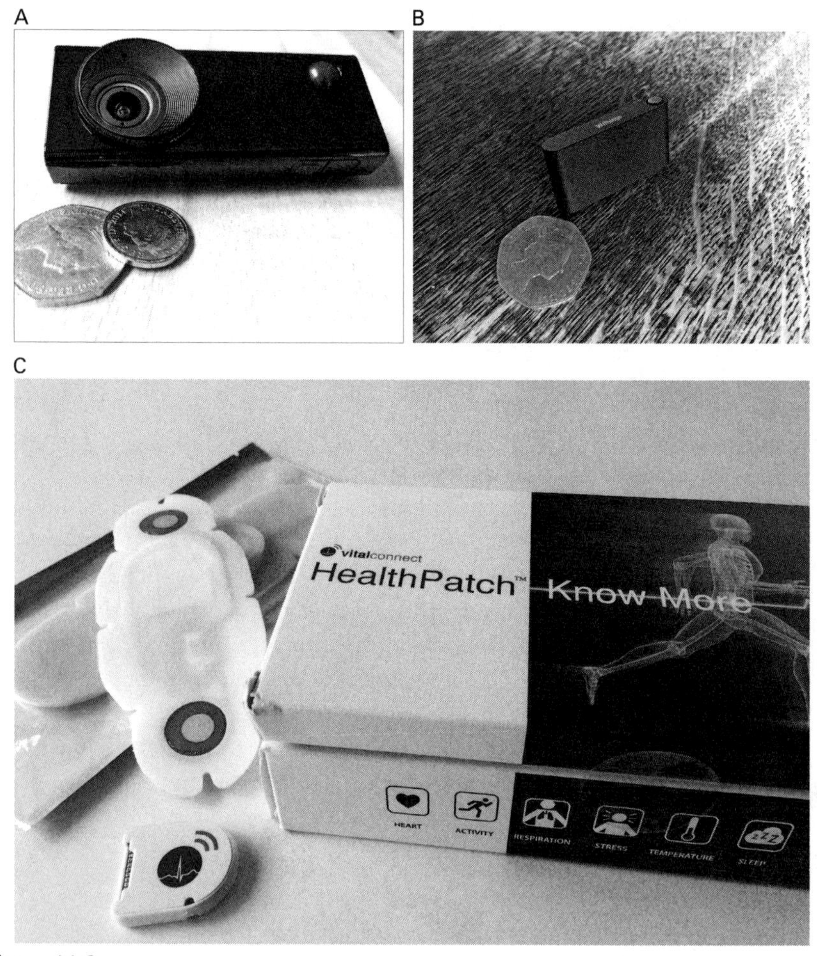


**Figure 11.2**
(a) Withings Pulse O2 activity tracker, (b) the Autographer, and (c) Vital Connects Health-Patch biosensor kit.

trails of bike flows. The cynically inclined would see the two docking stations at each end of my route as needed to fill the void between the glass-clad, elegant office blocks and high-rise apartment towers of Canary Wharf (to the south) and the heavily invested Stratford City (to the north). Both docking stations are in an area much like South East London that has so far not been on any plans to extend the bike rental scheme. During my forty-five-minute journey no activity is recorded at the Aberfeldy Street docking station while a total of 1,810 were completed across the network. In the week preceding my journey 18 journeys began from Aberfeldy Street against a seven-day total of 139,793 for the entire scheme. So the numbers show Aberfeldy Street's docking station to be at the quiet periphery of the rental scheme. Indeed, it's hard not to wonder how decisions are made about docking station locations and why out-of-the-way streets like Aberfeldy Street have them installed.

My aim then in starting off from Aberfeldy Street is to make room for sparse data, where the introduction of new mixtures of data might give us some clues to something else, something different. I want to avoid visualizing, yet again, the most common cycle journeys or where the flows are most dense (visualizations that seem to conveniently remind us where the wealth flows in London), and instead to see whether we might find other kinds of entangled relations.

So, taking the claims of difference surrounding data and (bio)sensing seriously, this is one shot at asking how the separations and associations might be cut differently, conforming not to long-established "regimes of existence," to borrow Genevieve Teil's (2012) evocative phrase, but, instead, offering up possibilities for refiguring the relational assemblies. The edges of the bike network, the introduction of bodily and geospatial and temporal data, are thus drawn together because of their capacities for change, for refiguring naturecultures. Although it may seem otherwise, this is a pragmatic quest. It is to begin thinking about data (with all its promise) as a real and material means of intervening in and disrupting the regimes. It is, as Karen Barad (2007) describes it, an attempt to participate in a responsive and responsible technoscience where the apparatus of scientific discovery (and more generally how we know things) are understood as means to make worlds, and thus also the means through which we might undo and remake them.

So, in closing, let me experiment with a way of recounting my bike ride and some of what surfaces along the way. In turning to the data, so to speak, I've picked out a moment that looks to me like one not of drama—of simultaneous peaks or troughs, or points of intersection—but where *the action* in the data appears to wane or dip (if only momentarily). I have sought out here the "caesura," as Paul Harrison (2002) calls it, not a point or span in the data where things add up or offer up some explanatory power, but where there seems to be no other way of judging it but as an exposure to the sensorium, of "that which incessantly, irretrievably, excessively, *happens*" (ibid., 490, emphasis in original).

Look then to 17:12 along the x-axis of the chart that follows (figure 11.3). There is a brief (~5mins) settling of my heart rate variability, seen in the denseness and relatively uniform swell of the dashed graph. The

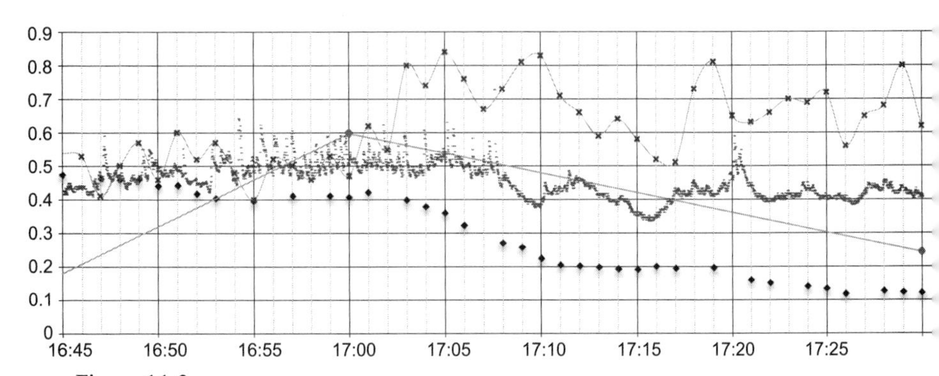


**Figure 11.3**
Graph of HRV levels (small dashes), rate of bike availability (diamonds), new bike rentals/100 (crosses), and body "activity" (dots).

number of bikes rented (cross markers) follows a not dissimilar curve. At the same time, the bike rate availability momentarily steadies with a flattening of the diamond markers—where (roughly) as many bikes are being taken from docking stations as being replaced.[7] What appeals to me in this narrow window onto three different data series is that the data don't "add up," they don't perform a story that coheres to what we know. Any correspondences between my biometric and bike data, especially, seem to be mere coincidence. The mutable moment of something like synchrony catches the eye, but at the same time the relations drift apart, forming connections that, if they exist at all, are a long way from anything we know.

Overlaying these data onto other kinds of data, this time geospatial, weaves yet longer unconnected/connected strands into this small window of time and space. Again, at 17:12, my ride intersects with an embankment running over the 150-year-old Northern Outfall Sewer, part of London's network of Victorian sewage systems (Lat 51°31'39.4435"N, Long 0°1'2.2544"E). Here, I move from the road to *The Greenway*, a raised foot and cycle path running about seven kilometers over sewage pipes and outlets between Bow and Beckton. Riding westward at 17:17 (as my momentary window falls away) and still on the Greenway, I catch sight of and find myself immediately north of the Abbey Mills pumping station (51°31'53.6"N 0°00'04.6"W), another still-operating monument to London's Victorian waterworks infrastructure (figure 11.4).

My five-minute ride then is over a very much living network, one that channels organic and molecular life, an effluent, smelt, intensely, in the air. The origins of the Northern Outfall Sewer and its tributaries channeling

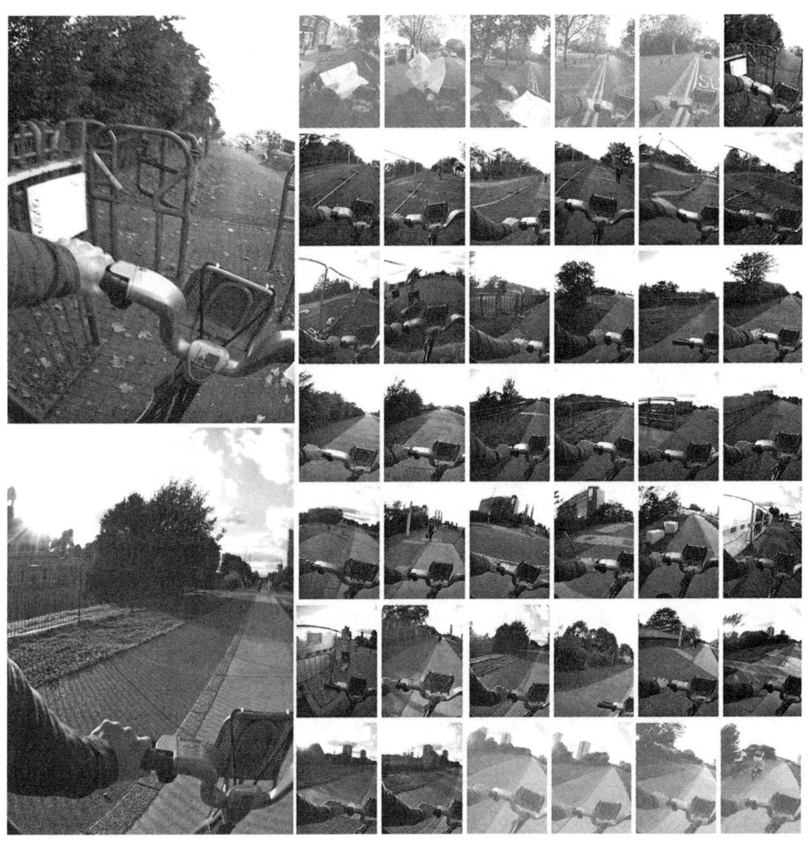

**Figure 11.4**
Autograph stream (right). Image from 17:12 (top left) and image from 17:17 (bottom left), with Abbey Mill pumping station to left, in sunlight.

this sewage are bound up with an economically vibrant London in the mid- to late 1800s, a city rapidly expanding due to its role as a major port and the massive industrialization of particular regions of the country. The Northern Outfall Sewer and its history also weaves into the cholera epidemics in London at the time and the acknowledged regulatory and political wrangling that put London's waterworks and drainage systems at the heart of the 1866 epidemic concentrated in the socially and economically deprived areas of East London (Halliday 2013). In 1886, the Abbey Mills pumping station was, originally, a temporary solution to pump low-level sewage into the Northern Outfall, with the express aim of at least partially sanitizing the water supply for those in the heavily affected areas of the east (ibid.).

And now, on and between these historic sewers, other kinds of infrastructural networks are taking shape. The bike rental scheme and divisive discussions about the directions of its planned expansion fold into the political atmosphere of contemporary London, where the politically conservative mayor is seeking to reduce the ever-spiraling costs of the city's transport system and at the same time reduce the proportion of public expenditure. Data here are of a kind that fits into a political/ideological and fiscal logic, where transport schemes (such as the rental bikes) are judged by their capital costs and the capacities they have for private investment (Hill 2014; Martin 2015). Also, this line drawn between my two coordinates of travel mark reconfigurations of a city's demographic, and the separations of wealth and poverty.

Looking east and south from the Greenway, you see aging housing stock, densely populated with first- or second-generation immigrant families mostly from South East Asia and a smattering of white communities carried over from a family ancestry in the docks and in itinerant factory and doss house work in the East End (wonderfully recorded by Orwell [1949]). Nested among the Victorian terraced houses, Green Street's market stalls and shops swell with life, people bustle among stalls and windows bright with gold jewelry, glittering saris and bridal ware, and colorful sweets, fruits, and vegetables. In contrast, "regeneration" to the north and west, symbolized by towering cranes and skeletal steel frames of buildings being built, is spurred on by heavy public-private investment—a legacy to the 2012 Olympics. Newham Council puts the levels of investment at £9billon so far,[8] but it's clear—looking from the raised embankment of the Greenway cutting through Newham—that much of this is concentrated to the northeast of the borough.

Amid the smells and Victorian network of tunnels, sewers and pumping stations, is then a dense mixture of pulsing mechanical and digital machines, bicycle and money flows, webs spun of human and political bodies, and, *in toto*, a city always already coming into being. The data continuously present/produced and brought together thickens things, it brings yet more life to a place. Above, is my experiment with cutting into this data phylum. The dips and flat lines in my own personally generated data etch new contours into the geography, ones intimately bound to place and time. Together, this spatio-temporal data may seem an odd mixture, one that mixes and matches unrelated ebbs and flows of stuff, worlds apart. Yet, at the same time they bring another kind of place to mind where past and present stories can be knitted into the land; recovered are the intermingling trajectories of hearts beating, lived lives, machines, infrastructural networks, spaces, times, politics, and so on. A body-in-place surfaces a panoply of data and relations, revealing the streams from "the hidden flows and their technological framing," drawing out, "the social relations and power mechanisms that are scripted in and enacted through these flows" (Kaika and Swyngedouw 2000, 121).

I want to say, to be clear, that my point here is not to make claims of any sort about how the data correlate, whether there are any right or wrong, or better or worse ways to slice through the aggregates. Rather, my interest is in how we can begin to work with the "speculative possibilities" (Sengers 2010, 22), how the data might suggest ways of doing things differently, and how we can start to ask different questions about and with the product of (bio)sensors—possibly more profound questions about the places we live in and how we live together.

## Other Worlds

Certainly one thing we might take away from these meanderings is that data structures and tools should be built to accommodate an expansion and thickening of worldly phenomena. The computational substrates that undergird the cloud and that are constitutive of big data should be given over to enlivening the relations, not flattening them. The trick here, as I see it, is to build in computational capacities that keep the vastness open, that don't slip too soon into neat classes—regimes even—of data that we know too well. Biosensing, self-tracking, and the like present the building blocks for such progressive capacities. Not merely ends in themselves—measuring things that many of us already have a sense of in/on our bodies—they are also the catalysts for discovering new relations between bodies all the way down (and up). And, this, it must be said, is big data's promise. There may still be little evidence of it, but the innovation in big data is precisely its potential for re-imagining relations. To return to boyd and Crawford, the "value comes from the patterns that can be derived by making connections" (boyd and Crawford 2011, 2). Big data's challenge is to take this challenge seriously.

Yet, there is more to it than this. The flux of data, bodies, places, and times—such as mine—provide us with a sense of a spatio-temporal phylum not just of what things *have* happened and the ways things are changing, but of how we might want them to be. The ever-thickening entanglements become possibilities for new cuts or planes. They are not merely where one *has* gone, but also a set of possibilities for how and where things can (or can't) materialize.

Alone, my own biosensed data does, of course, very little. My momentary slice, a caesura, through a space-time—triggered by some questions about biosensors, cycle flows, geographical coordinates, and so on—only hints at a vastness of traces through nodes and networks of past and present, and a multiplicity of options for moving on. But if we were to follow an open thread of "what ifs," might we just want to imagine what the (bio)sensed data produced from a much larger set of sources could do for us? Here we might take some speculative, tentative steps toward the possibilities of new worlds, of multiple worlds coming into being through relations just forming, new mixtures of Haraway's naturecultures that still need claiming, and that we can't yet know the knowings and beings they will enact.

My own inclination would be to see if and how the relations enacted might resist the strong forces at work in London, forces that prioritize regeneration over sustaining cultural life and tradition (Glucksberg 2014); that bypass or, worse still, erase the vibrancy of streets like Green Street in the uninvested areas of East London;[9] that literally build over the flows of effluence that have shaped a place and its people; that operate in and reinforce a city's pulse that orientates to the flows and rhythms of wealth and capital (Kaika 2014; Graham 2005). To my mind (and many others), these "agencies of homogenization" (Scott 1998) are figuring a cityscape that feels uniform, which masks and overwrites the unevenness and plurality that has made and makes London vibrant.

My question, then, would be to ask how (big) data might draw out the uneven and plural in the city, how, through (re-)figuring relations, we might begin to foreground the threads that weave through the multiple worlds that make up London rather than overlay them with a totalizing narrative that tidies and neatly compartmentalizes people and things. This is a data-sensing project that thrives on multiple worlds becoming. As I see it, it aims to locate (bio)sensed data within the ideas of "civility" and "conviviality" that Hinchliffe and Whatmore write of, ideas that concentrate our minds on "the practical intercorporeality of civic association in which particular kinds or individual entities thrive in combination with others whose capacities and powers enhance their own." (2006, 135). One might imagine that the data are used to tease out these productive combinations, algorithms that aren't just used to find intimate "soul mates" but also city-scale relations with those "capacities and powers" that exceed our own. Might our Boris Bikes move and brake in ways that resist some flows and aid others; might they afford new computationally constituted terrains in which our (bio)sensed rhythms ebb and flow unexpectedly; and, in the uncertain and unknown, might we discover combinations of difference that work?

And so my instrumented meanderings on a Boris Bike must stand as an experimental intervention aimed at opening questions. The bikes + data provide us with ways of imagining not merely a means to traverse the city, but also a means to etch out new surfaces, marking flows, momentary densities, gaps through time. Entangled in webs of (bio)sensors and worldly human/machine/political bodies, the data invite the space for something else. I find it hard to put it better than Nigel Thrift:

> We need spaces that graft. ... We need spaces that don't line up. We need spaces that breathe different atmospheres. We need new slopes, strips, roads, tracks, ridges, plains, seas. ... We need room. This is meant as an effort to make room. (Thrift 2014, 18)

## Notes

1. *Wired*, "The Petabyte Age: Because More Isn't Just More—More Is Different," June 23, 2008, Issue 16-07, http://archive.wired.com/science/discoveries/magazine/16-07/pb_intro, accessed August 25, 2015.

2. Vital Connect HealthPatch Biosensor, http://www.vitalconnect.com/health patch-biosensor, accessed August 13, 2015.

3. Privacy Policy Terms & Conditions, Vital Connect, Inc. Privacy Policy, January 1, 2013, http://www.vitalconnect.com./legal, accessed August 13, 2015.

4. Aventyn, "Digital Health: Interoperable Secure, Scalable with High-availability" (n.d), http://aventyn.com/Solutions.html, accessed August 13, 2015.

5. Heart rate variability (HRV) is the variation in the beat-to-beat interval of heartbeats.

6. The Autographer (now discontinued) is born of a project at my research laboratory in 2013. Presented in various guises, it has received considerable attention as a "memory augmentation" device, SenseCam. Purportedly, the streaming photos taken using SenseCam have been associated with improved memory recall for people suffering memory loss (Fleming 2014).

7. The data from the activity monitor (Withings Pulse O2) are only accessible for half-hour intervals, so it is of little use to the time-window considered here.

8. "Nine Billion Pounds of Private Investment in Stratford, Newham, Since the 2012 Games Were Announced," July 26, 2013, http://www.newham.gov.uk/Pages/News/Nine-billion-pounds-of-private-investment-in-Stratford,-Newham,-since-the-2012-gaames-were-announced.aspx, accessed August 13, 2015.

9. For a rich account of a similar street in London (in the south) see: Suzanne M. Hall, "Super-diverse Street: A 'Trans-Ethnography' across Migrant Localities," *Ethnic and Racial Studies* 38, no. 1 (2015): 22–37.

## References

Barad, K. 2007. *Meeting the Universe Halfway: Quantum Physics and the Entanglement of Matter and Meaning*. Chapel Hill, NC: Duke University Press.

Bowker, G. C. 2014. "Big Data, Big Questions: The Theory/Data Thing." *International Journal of Communication* 8 (5): 1795–1799.

boyd, d. and K. Crawford. 2011. "Six Provocations for Big Data." Paper presented at the symposium *A Decade in Internet Time: Symposium on the Dynamics of the Internet and Society*, 1–17. September. Oxford: Oxford Internet Institute.

Fleming, N. 2014. How Wearable Cameras Can Help Those with Alzheimer's. *The Guardian*. August 9. http://www.theguardian.com/technology/2014/aug/09/how-wearable-cameras-can-help-those-with-alzheimers. Accessed August 13, 2015.

Glucksberg, L. 2014. "'We Was Regenerated Out': Regeneration, Recycling and Devaluing Communities." *Valuation Studies* 2 (2): 97–118.

Graham, S. D. 2005. "Software-sorted Geographies." *Progress in Human Geography* 29 (5): 562–580.

Graham, S. D., and S. Marvin. 2001. *Splintering Urbanism: Networked Infrastructures, Technological Mobilities and the Urban Condition*. London: Routledge.

Halliday, S. 2013. *The Great Stink of London: Sir Joseph Bazalgette and the Cleansing of the Victorian Metropolis*. Stroud, Gloucestershire: The History Press.

Haraway, D. J. 1997. *Modest—Witness@ Second—Millennium. FemaleMan—Meets—OncoMouse: Feminism and Technoscience*. London: Routledge.

Haraway, D. J. 2003. *The Companion Species Manifesto: Dogs, People, and Significant Otherness*. vol. 1. Chicago: Prickly Paradigm Press.

Harrison, P. 2002. "The Caesura: Remarks on Wittgenstein's Interruption of Theory, or, Why Practices Elude Explanation." *Geoforum* 33 (4): 487–503.

Hill, D. 2014. "The Great Boris Bus Stop." *The Guardian*. August 30. http://www.theguardian.com/uk-news/davehillblog/2014/aug/30/the-great-boris-bus-stop. Accessed August 13, 2015.

Hinchliffe, S., and S. Whatmore. 2006. "Living Cities: Towards a Politics of Conviviality." *Science as Culture* 15 (2): 123–138.

Kaika, M. 2014. "The Uncanny Materialities of the Everyday." In *Infrastructural Lives: Urban Infrastructure in Context*, ed. S. Graham and C. McFarlane, 139–152. London: Routledge.

Kaika, M., and E. Swyngedouw. 2000. "Fetishizing the Modern City: The Phantasmagoria of Urban Technological Networks." *International Journal of Urban and Regional Research* 24 (1): 120–138.

Kitchin, R. 2014. "Big Data, New Epistemologies and Paradigm Shifts." *Big Data & Society* 1 (1). http://bds.sagepub.com/content/1/1/2053951714528481.short. Accessed August 13, 2015.

Lindley, S. E., C. C. Marshall, R. Banks, A. Sellen, and T. Regan. 2013. "Rethinking the Web as a Personal Archive." In *Proceedings of the 22nd International Conference on World Wide Web*, 749–760. May. Republic and Canton of Geneva, Switzerland: International World Wide Web Conferences Steering Committee.

Martin, I. 2015. "The City that Privatised Itself to Death: 'London Is Now a Set of Improbable Sex Toys Poking Gormlessly into the Air.'" *The Guardian*. February 24. http://www.theguardian.com/politics/2015/feb/24/the-city-that-privatised-itself-to-death-london-is-now-a-set-of-improbable-sex-toys-poking-gormlessly-into-the-air. Accessed August 13, 2015.

O'Brien, O. 2014. "From Putney to Poplar: 12 Million Journeys on the London Bikeshare." September 11. http://oobrien.com/2014/09/from-putney-to-poplar-12-million-journeys-on-the-london-bikeshare/. Accessed August 13, 2015.

Orwell, G. 1949. *Down and Out in London and Paris*. London: Penguin Books.

Scott, J. C. 1998. *Seeing Like a State: How Certain Schemes to Improve the Human Condition Have Failed*. New Haven, CT, and London: Yale University Press.

Sengers, I. 2010. "Including the Nonhuman in Political Theory: Opening Pandora's Box." In *Political Matter*, ed. B. Braun and S. J. Whatmore, 3–33. Minneapolis, Minnesota: University of Minnesota Press.

Shklovski, I., S. D. Mainwaring, H. H. Skúladóttir, and H. Borgthorsson. 2014. "Leakiness and Creepiness in App Space: Perceptions of Privacy and Mobile App Use." In *Proceedings of the 32nd Annual ACM Conference on Human Factors in Computing Systems*, 2347–2356. April. New York: ACM.

Short, A. 2011. "TfL's Information Doesn't Want to Be Free." January 7. https://adrianshort.org/tfls-information-doesnt-want-to-be-free/. Accessed August 13, 2015.

Siddle, J. 2014. "London Maps and Bike Rental Communities, According to Boris Bike Journey Data." March 2. http://vartree.blogspot.co.uk/2014/03/london-maps-and-bike-rental-communities.html. Accessed August 13, 2015.

Star, S. L., and A. Strauss. 1999. "Layers of Silence, Arenas of Voice: The Ecology of Visible and Invisible Work." *Computer Supported Cooperative Work* 8 (1–2): 9–30.

Teil, G. 2012. "No Such Thing as Terroir? Objectivities and the Regimes of Existence of Objects." *Science, Technology & Human Values* 37 (5): 478–505.

Thrift, N. 2014. "The 'Sentient' City and What It May Portend." *Big Data & Society* 1(1). http://bds.sagepub.com/content/1/1/2053951714532241.short. Accessed August 13, 2015.

Wilson, M. W. 2011. "Data Matter(s): Legitimacy, Coding, and Qualifications-of-Life." *Environment and Planning. D, Society & Space* 29 (5): 857–872.

# 12

# The Data Citizen, the Quantified Self, and Personal Genomics

Judith Gregory and Geoffrey C. Bowker

The rise of the quantified self and personal social genomics movements pose fundamental questions about the nature of citizenship that go well beyond the confines of reductive concepts of privacy. As we live more and more algorithmically through self-tracking, our identities are necessarily being caught up in the cloud.

## Introduction: We Are All "Data Citizens"

In 1941, pragmatist philosopher Arthur F. Bentley wrote a classic essay entitled: "The Human Skin: Philosophy's Last Line of Defense," where he argued that it was epistemologically absurd to separate off the knower (inside the skin) and the known (outside the skin) (Bentley 1941). Rather, he said, we should look at knower and known from the point of view of the knower-known system as a whole.

We argue that seeing the citizen in there (beneath the naked skin) and data about the citizen out there (circulating within ever denser industrial and governmental networks) is equally misconceived; it is thus an instance of misplaced concretism[1] (Whitehead 1925 [1919], Whitehead 1997 [1925][2]; Wildman and Michelson 1969 [1967]; Hickman and Spadafora 2009; Star 1994) which leads us to a raft of concepts (such as privacy) that inevitably wind up in aporias. We maintain that by looking integrally at the "data citizen" we can move beyond these and begin to construct a viable ethics for our brave new world.

The argument follows in three parts. First, we motivate the concept of the data citizen and its policy relevance. Second, taking the lens of the quantified self and personal genomics we discuss five settings in which we can discern the data citizen in action. Third, and finally, we draw up some policy recommendations and design principles derived from this move.

## Insides and Outsides

It is commonplace today to deny the centrality of the skin in human biology. While "the skin" definitely has a role ("keeping your insides in" as Allan Sherman remarked[3]), it is clear that we are not the sum total of our genetic information. We are at birth bequeathed microflora and microfauna, which at the end of the day constitute 90 percent of the cells in our bodies—these microbiomes within which and together with "we" live affect our physical and psychological health, tailored only in some ways to ourselves. Further, we are integrally part of wider communities both within and without: our exposome encompasses not only our personal genome and the flora and fauna that inhabit our personal living spaces but also all "life-course environmental exposures (including lifestyle factors), from the prenatal period onwards" (Wild 2005).

If we see ourselves as basically elucidated by the information in our DNA, then it becomes extremely difficult to account for this community of self within which we live and through which we live together. And it becomes difficult to work out good biodiversity policy—for example, if we reify species (a misplaced concretism excoriated in the philosophy of biology) into independent entities that can be somehow independently stored and saved (in seed banks, or in silico) then we are necessarily missing the point of the nature of life on earth and end up saving the wrong kinds of units, elements, beings. These may be human-nonhuman collectives and/or individual and familial life trajectories that are culturally patterned and locative. Taking the relationship as ontologically prior (Bowker 2014) rather than the entity, we not only understand the world differently, but we also interact with it in different ways.

## Toward a Policy Process on What Data to Share and How

There is a close analogy here with the role of data in our lives. We live in the epoch of the database (Manovich 1998, 2013; Bowker 2013). From birth, we are measured, described, and both acted upon and partially constituted by these circulating data. We are in a *recurso* that goes back to the period of the Enlightenment, when the first great national censuses were brought into being, along with and enabling the first great epidemiological surveys. Together, they gave us data about social circumstances and our health, which in turn affected our lives both directly—personally—and through the development of policy related to such data (childhood nutritional programs, health screening, and more). Large-scale systematic data collection moved our being into complex information networks that constitute our selves and our society. There is great uncertainty about what data to share and how, for which we need to conceptualize and iteratively evolve a policy process.

What happens when you try to keep the "insides" in is demonstrated by the birth and death of the concept of privacy in the home. Privacy law over the past thirty years has dealt uneasily with this concretization of the concept. Is your car an extension of your home such that what is in there is under the same protection? Is your cell phone—password protected or not—geographically located (part of your office) or should it be searchable if you are stopped?[4] Indeed, privacy as often conceived in policy circles is largely an empty concept, when data pooling and data analytics together render as moot the whole idea of what is inside and therefore protected. There are not enough locks in the world to keep data from talking with each other. And many are the proofs that locking personal data within a virtual box with metadata inscribed on its envelope is similarly misconceived (see, e.g., Harvard[5]); "Metadata is not just 'the envelope' rather than its contents."[6]

Consider the (idealized) phenomenology of the citizen of the modern state. Performative data streams begin to circulate out of the unformed fetus. If the fetus has girl potential, it may in certain cultures be cut off before birth. If the fetus is suffering from Down's syndrome, it may not be allowed into the world of the working healthy—and if it is, the child will circulate from birth along predetermined social and medical channels. Once born, he or she is given a gender (forcibly in the case of the intersexed, for we live in a world of binary data that are entered into population statistics—along with data about ethnicity and health). Increasingly from birth, her/his genetic data are stored by governmental agencies for medical and/or other monitoring—policing—purposes; in both cases arguably for her/his later protection, though this is always the underlying rationale for attacks on privacy. Barely out of her/his mother's womb, data are circulating out of her/him into agencies that transform the data and produce actions and policies and practices that come back to act upon and within her/him. Just as she/he was born with an ecology of microflora and microfauna, so is she/he born into an ecology of microdata. Both ecologies are performative. For the microdata, at the large scale, they help shape social policy that affects her/his living conditions; at smaller scales, they trigger a set of responses that affect her/his daily life and the lives of those nearby whether by family, social circles or "common fate"[7] following theorists of Gestalt principles. And she/he is barely out of the womb. ... To imagine a "citizen" as an ideal type who exists outside of data flows is then conceptually flawed: she/

he becomes a citizen because she/he is saturated by data flows, markers, indicators, analyses. Later in life, few will be forks in her/his path that are not modulated by (note we are not saying "determined by") these data flows—recommender systems will with increasing accuracy channel her/his and her/his consorts into sets of interests which render her/him and them as integrally good consumers and contented—if not satisfied—ones. The question with data is not *whether* data are essential, will circulate, will be used—but *how* so.

Taken together, the quantified self (QS) social identity and self-tracking movement and, in parallel, the rise of personal genomics can be seen as recognition and problematic appropriation of this data ecology. The future imaginary of the QS movement is that the QS data citizen will be able to live her/his life to the fullest through being optimally fit physically, cognitively, and emotionally in order to be the best person, worker, leader, and consumer she/he can be. It seems that we are moving into a brave new world, but once we look beyond the resplendence of modern techniques of personal quantification, this can be seen, again, as an essential dimension of the epoch of the database. Fifty years ago, measures were generally more circumscribed in their travels and fewer. We measured our temperature against an ideal number (98.4F) to know if we were running a fever. As children, our parents tracked our height, often by notches on a doorpost. One of our great modern obsessions, our body mass index (BMI), was first calculated by the great social statistician Adolphe Quételet in the early nineteenth century (Quételet 1869). Another obsession, calorie counting, began in the early twentieth century (see, e.g., Schüll 2012). What is fundamentally different about the modern form of QS is that its data have begun to flow into precisely the same kinds of channels—medical, commercial, governmental—that we have just described. The data from our devices—be they glasses, watches, tattoos on the skin, or woven into "smart" clothes—are uploaded onto websites so that we can finetune our bodies and minds to ideal numbers, and so that these data may be used to design ever more applications (hereafter "apps"), gadgets, devices—and to share our data with agencies and entities that seek to influence us.

## The Design/Policy Knot

The policy issues that arise from QS and like movements cannot be addressed by assuming that we may exist outside of our data flows. We maintain, following Jackson, Gillespie, and Payette (2014) that fundamentally we are dealing with a *design/policy knot*. Thinking of the design/

policy knot indicates that it's not about producing universal principles, but about looking for and nurturing an ongoing process. You cannot design a data system and *then* look at its policy implications—you're already too late. Inversely, you cannot state a policy apodictically and then design technology to suit: every policy enshrined in a concept of a citizen "out there" beyond data misses the performative point that what it is to be a citizen and what it is to be a person bring us to the possibility of being a new kind of data citizen. Every such policy, then, is fundamentally affected by the very design of our data flows and the social and engineering technologies that constitute our data ecologies.

We take up the Quantified Self and personal genomics social movements as microcosms for considering contexts and practices of and in relation to biosciences and biosensors, and how they inform our thinking about becoming data citizens and concepts of data citizenship. At the end of the day, we are especially interested in altruism, reciprocity, and immanence in this our brave new world.

## Quantified Selves and Personal Genomics: Bioscience, Biosensors, Contexts, and Practices

The pervasive social trend now known as "the Quantified Self movement" orients toward self-tracking health and activity—also known as person-generated data—by means of wearable and other devices, apps, social media-oriented websites, and other sites and sources of digitally available health data via mobile phone or on the web. In the Health Data Exploration Project in which we participated (Health Data Exploration Project 2014;[8] see also http://www.rwjf.org/en/library/research/2014/03/personal-data-for-the-public-good.html, accessed August 20, 2015), a surprising result was the marked willingness of individuals to share their personal data with other parties—even in many cases non-anonymously—for the public good.

Willingness and intentions for broader kinds of sharing are expressed particularly in regard to personal genomics.[9] As examples among many: the "Million Veteran" campaign by the U.S. Veterans Affairs Office of Research and Development for donations of blood samples for genomics analysis (that will be anonymized); the gift of data from 100,000 member-patients of the U.S. health-care company Kaiser Permanente (a nonprofit trust) in conjunction with the University of California–San Francisco Institute for Human Genetics with support from the National Institutes of Health (https://www.ucsf.edu/news/2011/07/10305/ucsf-and

-kaiser-permanente-complete-massive-genotyping-project); and the Personal Genome Project in which each contributor can modulate degrees of anonymity and sharing along a scale that includes the option of sharing in an open data commons (see, e.g., Angrist 2009).[10]

How may novel technologies and new kinds of personal data contribute to the public good, as a positively "disruptive" turning point that could provoke new modes of agency of individuals in their health, health and biomedical sciences research, and new kinds of "data commons" in which citizens and researchers can contribute and share data? How and why are people willing to share data about themselves? Table 12.1 outlines some possible parameters people might use in thinking through this question. How may new kinds of research collaboration be fostered—for example among "dream teams" that invite citizen participation—that could bring together multidisciplinary biomedical, health, policy, and social sciences researchers with companies and communities that design and make apps, devices, websites, and platforms, and thus hold self-tracked data generated by individuals and collectives? Under what kinds of governance and circumstances might companies make available the data they collect from individuals, might researchers make use of self-tracked data in their research, and might individuals be willing to share their data? Do we need "a new Belmont Report" (NCPHS 1979)—the current gold standard of ethics principles—to address the privacy, confidentiality, and anonymity of personal data in this brave new era? And if so, through what kind of a process will we develop it?

In self-identified Quantified Self meet-ups, there's often a first-person narrative mode formatted as: What did I/we do? How did I/we do it? What did I/we learn? Personal narratives of self-quantification and knowledge gained by quantification and analysis over time and their visualization are proliferating. Yet some recent findings indicated that there might not be as much sharing of QS data as we think, even though in principle there is a willingness to do so (see, e.g., Health Data Exploration Project 2014). Concurrently, there is much sharing that occurs 1:1 in intimate relationships and sharing, much data tracking that is done on behalf of another person, much quantitative "registration" kept for regular routines (e.g., daily) of the body that are not written down but "only kept in the head," much handwritten recordkeeping related to long-term clinical care, medication regimes, or for physical, cognitive, or medical recovery, whether for an acute condition or life-long (see Fox and Duggan 2013).

The theoretical link with data citizenship/data governance is that people don't have a good grasp about how their data can, will, and perhaps

**Table 12.1**
Willingness to Share Quantified Self Data in Scientific Research

| | |
|---|---|
| ACCESS: Respondent wants to be able to access his/her own data or the entire dataset as well. | NO GOVERNMENT: Data must not be used by the government. |
| AGGREGATE: Researchers can only have access to aggregated data or only report in the aggregate. This is closely related to privacy. | NON-COMMERCIAL: Non-commercial or nonprofit research only. |
| BENEFIT: Respondent should benefit in some way from the research (non-monetary). | OPT OUT: Respondent must be able to opt out of the study. |
| DEPENDS: General "It depends" statements. | OWNERSHIP: Respondent must retain ownership/control of data. |
| DEPENDS/DATA: It depends on the data. In other words, the respondent would be more willing to share some data than other data. | PAID: Monetary or similar compensation. |
| FEEDBACK: Researchers must return results of the study to the participants. | PRIVACY: Must protect/assure privacy of participants. This includes any mention of a privacy requirement, even if not absolute. Key terms included here are "privacy," "private," anonymous," "confidential," "do not want my named attached." |
| GREATER GOOD: Research must be for the greater good, e.g.: "If there is definitely a benefit for the greater good, i.e. to help address a disease, etc." | PROTECTION: Data cannot be used to discriminate against or deny service to Respondent. This includes use by insurance companies to set rates or deny coverage, use by employers in hiring, etc. |
| INFORMED: Respondent wants to be informed about the particular study or purpose of the research. Implies no general-purpose databases. | REPUTATION: Respondent would only share data with trusted researchers or institutions. |
| IRB/HIPAA: Specific mention of IRB, HIPAA, or similar regulatory mechanism. | RESEARCH: Data can only be used for research studies, not for marketing, product development, etc. |
| LOVED ONE: Would only share data if it would directly benefit a loved one. | RESTITUTION: Respondent wants to be able to get restitution for data misuse. |
| NO ADDS: No advertising or market research purposes. | TIME LIMIT: Data shared only for finite, specified time. |
| NO CONDITIONS: Would share freely without any conditions. | TRUST COMPANY: Respondent would only allow sharing if he/she trusted the company that held his/her data. |
| NO EFFORT: Sharing data for research must not require extra effort for the respondent. | WOULD NOT: Respondent would not share his/her data regardless of condition. |

Source: Non-published preliminary data depiction (2013). Courtesy of the Health Data Exploration Project, University of California-San Diego and University of California-Irvine. M. J. Bietz, G. C. Bowker, S. Calvert, M. Claffey, J. Gregory, A. Hubenko, K. Patrick, R. Rao, and J. Sheehen. For the published report, see Personal Data for the Public Good: New Opportunities to Enrich Understanding of Individual and Population Health, Health Data Exploration Project, 2014. Supported by the Robert Wood Johnson Foundation.

should be used. As in the "privacy paradox" (Norberg, Horne, and Horne 2007), when you ask people if they care about data, they say they do. If you look at their practices, many actually don't interact with their data very much or very often. That's why we need to understand practices, not only expressed opinions, to get at what people are actually doing. By the same token, we need better empirical understanding of people's relationship to their own data as a rich field to study from the design angle (how to turn caring into doing) and from the social angle (understanding what issues are at stake for the citizens of tomorrow).

### The Data Citizen Project: New Forms of Data Work of the Self and in Personal Life

Deeper understandings of living algorithmically individually and collectively through sharing self-tracking and personal genomics data in quantifying communities are also about our relationships with data about our selves. New kinds of data require new kinds of data citizens engaging in policy debates about the collection and deployment of these large new datasets, together exploring—with the wider publics—the social, cultural, and ethical issues arising in these vast data collection enterprises.

A variety of discourses concern how novel technologies and new kinds of personal data may contribute to the public good, as a positively "disruptive" turning point that could provoke new modes of agency of individuals in their health, health and biomedical sciences research, and new kinds of data commons in which citizens and researchers can contribute and share data. For these to come about, we need a critical approach to "genetic empowerment" as well as public understandings of as yet invisible algorithms. The mantra for "P4 Medicine" is for genetic empowerment to be "predictive, preventive, personalized, and participatory" (Hood and Galas 2003). Challenging questions abound: What role will personal genetics play in clinical dynamics? What do data citizens want to know? How will "fear of genetic fate" (ibid.) be addressed?

A growth area in QS is the relatively new availability of personal genomic testing. For example, for less than $100 companies like 23andMe will provide a kit for customers to send in a DNA sample that is then analyzed for approximately 250 aspects of health from back pain to breast cancer. Similarly, metagenomic analysis (genomic testing of populations of microorganisms) is being offered as a way to understand the ecosystem of nonhuman organisms to which our bodies play host. There is a growing awareness within the QS community and beyond (see chapter 1, this volume) that personal information can be even more powerful when it is made social. Several QS citizen science projects have started to aggregate personal genomic and metagenomic data to, for example, "publish their test results, find others with similar genetic variations, learn more about their results, find the latest primary literature on their variations and help scientists to find new associations."[11] As a commonplace yet profound change, sleep research is exemplary in the transformation of knowledge enabled by digital wearables by the change from being sequestered in special cocoons to being in one's natural habitat at home.

There is profound potential to lead new kinds of research, sciences, and caring practices, yet there are policy lacunae in regard to consumers' everyday practices of routinely signing off on "terms and conditions"—as the condition for use of a services, an app, site, device, or gadget. Terms and conditions for big data services (QS, social media) more and more grant corporate ownership, use, reuse, and sale of users' data corpus in part or in whole to other companies (as an integral part of the companies' business models), whereas the individual human user-owner-subscriber(s) of the gadget or digital service might not have full rights or co-ownership to his or her own "raw" data stream (having routinely signed off rights to the self-generated data).[12] These matters of concern are coming onto the public and policy radar (see especially Health Data Exploration Project 2014).

From research perspectives, we are especially interested in how new kinds of research practices and collaborations may be fostered. We see potential for "dream teams" that could bring together multidisciplinary biomedical, health, and social sciences researchers with companies that design devices, apps, websites, and platforms and thus hold self-tracked data generated by individuals. In regard to quantified selves and personal genomics, there is a much tighter connection from the beginning in policy, design, and practice, with policy not yet relevant enough to the kinds of infrastructures that we already have and that are evolving around us. Because social practices have their own autonomies in sense making, rhythms, commitments, disparate and consonant logics, and temporalities, there is a quickening and tightening up of interweaving in relation to health, biosciences, biosensors, and bioscience technologies—a need for more dynamic knowledge infrastructures (Edwards et al. 2013).

A "design/policy knot" ties together policy, design, and practice. They ravel, unravel, and ravel again and over time. We can tie together a design/policy knot with the development of new kinds of dream teams, ones that must include designers integrally with policy makers as an ongoing principle of governance (i.e., not as a one-off moment). The problem for most ethics frameworks (e.g., the Belmont Report, 1979) are that they are seldom or never modified but rather conceived as "standing the test of time." Yet technology is changing so fast in these interlaced arenas that there is no possible set of universal principles that transcends the technology since we are *constituted* differently as data citizens at different technological moments. Thus a dream team can become a form that engages an "ideal" yet "materially" grounded iterative process.

## Thinking about Design: Knowledge through the Senses, Poetics, Reflection

Personal genomics communities and communities such as QS can develop and extend sharing practices in regard to health, wellness, and sharing and caring practices, augmenting established sites such as the PatientsLikeMe, rare illnesses groups, and Pharmville, creating more intimate or more open spaces.

We consider personal genomics at five scales:

1. one's past, present, future
2. one's self, family, ancestors, and the future
3. one's genes, one's markers, one's health
4. data big and small, innately intimate data
5. the social, the cultural, new communities

For each we offer a haiku to express these condensed essences of phenomenal layers.

Haiku for Scale 1: one's past, present, future

**The Normal and the Pathological**[13]

Alleles jump and switch and change places
Passenger and driver
Context is everything

Haiku for Scale 2: one's self, family, ancestors, and the future

**Unexpected Utopias Alongside Dystopias**

It never occurred to me
That this could become
About undoing stigma

Haiku for Scale 3: one's genes, one's markers, one's health

**Transformations of Knowledge**

Genomics bio-mantra
Predictive, proactive
Preventive—but not always

Haiku for Scale 4: data big and small, innately intimate data

**Corporeal and Corporate Landscapes**

Personal genomics
Are all at once ancestral
Temporally back and forth

Haiku for Scale 5: the social, the cultural, new communities

**Altruism and Reciprocity**

Walking our cities
One million veterans
Framingham renews

And a sixth Haiku: on knowledge transformations, things falling apart and coming together anew

Science spins 360°
Reversals, re-births
Of scientific knowledge[14]

## Interlude

In "Self Help," poet Katie Peterson refracts her verse on the metamorphosis of the mind:

The eye is the lamp of the body so I tried to make a world where all I ate was light. Butterflies complete a similar labor in the summer garden, beating their wings slowly like a healthy person, the kind of person who runs for fun, could run from an attacker, eats greens in the same quantity as the salty meats the storytelling part of us appears to favor. I couldn't decide whether I wanted to stay alive or wanted to go faster, they appeared to contradict each other, I tried in all I did to eat light. I left the argument about the difference between a slave and a servant on the table though I think what I think is that consent to servitude is as much fiction as a butterfly having a nervous breakdown because of the beauty of the lavender. The longer your hunger takes to find a shape the longer you can hold it. Consider the butterfly, only at rest in the middle of consumption, but even then practicing for departure, for disappearance, closing in the middle of the landscape. Trying to manage a world in which all you can eat is light is difficult. Labor, and the lungs should be like wings of the butterfly beating, closing, slowly, the moonlight tensing the edge of each, almost lifting the edge of each towards the middle distance. So all that I consume can make me healthy, illuminate my throat and the interstate of my digestive tract with what a butterfly's been swimming in" (Deacon and Peterson 2014).

## Concluding Thoughts

On the entrepreneurial side, companies both large and small, established and startups, need to build in consumers' privacy protections at every stage in developing their products. A more expansive notion of data citizenship might suggest to companies the possibility of considering forms of co-ownership with the people who use and elaborate their digital offerings. These could be reasonable security for consumer data, limited collection and retention of such data, and reasonable procedures to promote data accuracy (see FTC 2010). Here, too, practices run ahead of policy and visions for shared horizons.

If the notion of the "data citizen" suggests that data are always, in a sense, already "shared," then there is also a vast opportunity to create design spaces for individuals, social circles, health and medical fields, biosciences, scientific discovery. This design for novel design spaces could consider, but not be limited to, cross-sensory surrounds and affordances such as synesthesia (Deacon and Peterson 2014, 122), artful abstraction (Dickerman 2013 [2012]), visual elegance and visible language, aural sensation and subtleties of sound, the tactile, the poetic, interactive vignettes that can be personalized, tales from the future, epistolary and otherwise, mindfulness, restfulness, peacefulness, wisdom-enhancing. In brief, the conditions of possibility exist to design for new digital literacies in shared data.

We end as we began with our belief and hope in altruism, reciprocity, and immanence.

## Acknowledgments

We wish especially to acknowledge Matthew J. Bietz, Tom Boellstorff, Paul Dourish, John E. Mattison, Dawn Nafus, Helen Nissenbaum, and Katherine Pine among many more inspired and inspiring colleagues than we can count. We wish to thank the Intel Science & Technology Center on Social Computing for supporting our preliminary study "An Exploratory Study of Personal Genomics and Metagenomics in the Quantified Self Movement" with a seed grant in relation to the research themes *Algorithmic Living* and *Information Ecosystems*.

## Notes

1. On concretism, see http://www.finedictionary.com/concretism.html, accessed August 20, 2015.

2. Alfred North Whitehead posited the *fallacy of misplaced concreteness* as when one mistakes an abstract belief, opinion, or concept about the way things are for a physical or "concrete" reality: "There is an error; but it is merely the accidental error of mistaking the abstract for the concrete. It is an example of what I

will call the 'Fallacy of Misplaced Concreteness'" (Whitehead 1997 [1925], 51). Whitehead proposed the fallacy in a discussion of the relation of spatial and temporal location of objects. He argued: "among the primary elements of nature as apprehended in our immediate experience, there is no element whatever which possesses this character of simple location. ... Accordingly, the real error is an example of what I have termed: The Fallacy of Misplaced Concreteness" (Whitehead 1925 [1919]).

3. https://www.youtube.com/watch?v=mZI12WHWvAg, accessed August 20, 2015.

4. See, e.g., the U.S. Supreme Court ruling at time of writing: http://www.nytimes.com/2014/06/26/us/supreme-court-cellphones-search-privacy.html, accessed August 18, 2015.

5. E-Mail Management: Guide for Harvard Administrators, Records Management Services, Harvard University Archives, http://library.harvard.edu/sites/default/files/E-MailManagementAGuideForHarvardAdministrators_0.pdf, accessed August 20, 2015.

6. http://www.cnet.com/news/what-you-need-to-know-about-data-retention/, accessed August 20, 2015; http://www.voidynullness.net/blog/2015/03/03/definition-of-metadata-mass-surveillance/, accessed July 30, 2015.

7. See, e.g., http://en.wikipedia.org/wiki/Principles_of_grouping#Common_Fate, accessed August 20, 2015: "When visual elements are seen moving in the same direction at the same rate (optical flow), perception associates the movement as part of the same stimulus. For example, birds may be distinguished from their background as a single flock because they are moving in the same direction and at the same velocity, even when each bird is seen—from a distance—as little more than a dot. The moving 'dots' appear to be part of a unified whole. Similarly, two flocks of birds can cross each other in a viewer's visual field, but they will nonetheless continue to be experienced as separate flocks because each bird has a direction common to its flock. This allows people to make out moving objects even when other details (such as the object's color or outline) are obscured. This ability likely arose from the evolutionary need to distinguish a camouflaged predator from its background. The law of common fate is used extensively in user-interface design, for example ... [t]he movement of a physical mouse is synchronized with the movement of an on-screen arrow cursor, and so on."

8. We wish to acknowledge the Robert Wood Johnson Foundation for support to the Health Data Exploration Project.

9. Both by avant-garde groups such as the Personal Genome Project and evidenced by public enrollments in donating.

10. The Personal Genome Project (PGP) has the most interesting informed consent process that one of the authors has experienced in that (a) the PGP Genome-Wide Association (GWA) should not be a donor's first encounter with one's personal genomics, that is to say the donor must have some self-knowledge about his or her genetic information via 23andMe, clinically or otherwise; (b) to contribute data from one's GWA, you must read some pages on the basic science of genomics and pass a test as assurance that you understand basic principles and

terms of genomics; (c) the consent explanations are explicit about the uncertain and changing state of personal genomics knowledge; and (d) the consent process is iterative in consideration of new knowledge discovery that may change understandings.

11. http://opensnp.org, accessed August 20, 2015; see also Personal Genome Project at http://www.personalgenomes.org, accessed August 20, 2015.

12. Policy lacunae on terms and conditions were evident in a recent national science policy discussion yet blind to this.

13. Canguilhem (1991). The Normal and the Pathological, with an introduction by Michel Foucault. New York: Zone Books.

14. Referencing "Russ Altman's Translational Biomedical Informatics Year in Review" (Altman 2011–2014).

## References

Altman, Russ B. 2011. "Translational Bioinformatics 2011: The Year in Review." https://dl.dropboxusercontent.com/u/2734365/amia-tb-review-11.pdf. Accessed August 18, 2015.

Altman, Russ B. 2012. "Translational Bioinformatics 2012 Year in Review." https://rbaltman.wordpress.com/2012/03/22/translational-bioinformatics-2012-year-in-review/. Accessed August 18, 2015.

Altman, Russ B. 2013. "Translational Bioinformatics Year in Review 2013." https://rbaltman.wordpress.com/2013/03/21/materials-from-translational-bioinformatics-year-in-review-2013. Accessed August 18, 2015.

Altman, Russ B. 2014. "Russ Altman's Translational Biomedical Informatics Year in Review." http://gettinggeneticsdone.blogspot.com/2014/04/russ-altmans-translational.html. Accessed August 18, 2015.

Angrist, Misha. 2009. "Eyes Wide Open: the Personal Genome Project: Citizen Science and Veracity in Informed Consent." Per Med. Nov. 6 (6): 691–699.

Bentley, Arthur F. 1941. "The Human Skin: Philosophy's Last Line of Defense." *Philosophy of Science* 8:1–19.

Bowker, Geoffrey C. 2013. "Data Flakes: An Afterword to *'Raw Data' Is an Oxymoron*." In *"Raw Data" Is an Oxymoron*, ed. Lisa Gitelman, 167–171. Cambridge, MA: MIT Press.

Bowker, Geoffrey C. 2014. "The Theory/Data Thing." *International Journal of Communication* 8:1795–1799.

Canguilhem, Georges. 1991. *The Normal and the Pathological*. With an introduction by Michel Foucault. New York: Zone Books.

Deacon, Richard, and Katie Peterson. 2014. "Sensory Perception: A Picture and a Poem." *The New York Times Style Magazine*. http://tmagazine.blogs.nytimes.com/2014/04/03/a-picture-and-a-poem-sensory-perception/?_r=0. Accessed April 14, 2015.

Dickerman, Leah. 2013 [2012]. *Inventing Abstraction, 1910–1925: How a Radical Idea Changed Modern Art.* 2nd printing. New York: The Museum of Modern Art.

Edwards, Paul N., Stephen J. Jackson, Melissa K. Chalmers, Geoffrey C. Bowker, Christine L. Borgman, David Ribes, and Scout Calvert. 2013. "Knowledge Infrastructures: Intellectual Frameworks and Research Challenges." Report of a workshop sponsored by the National Science Foundation and the Sloan Foundation, University of Michigan School of Information, Ann Arbor, May 25–28, 2012. http://deepblue.lib.umich.edu/handle/2027.42/97552. Accessed August 18, 2015.

Federal Trade Commision. 2010. "Protecting Consumer Privacy in an Era of Rapid Change." https://www.ftc.gov/sites/default/files/documents/reports/federal-trade-commission-bureau-consumer-protection-preliminary-ftc-staff-report-protecting-consumer/101201privacyreport.pdf. Accessed August 18, 2015.

Fox, Susannah, and Maeve Duggan. 2013. "Tracking for Health." Pew Internet & American Life Project. http://www.pewinternet.org/2013/01/28/tracking-for-health/. Accessed August 18, 2015.

Health Data Exploration Project. 2014. Personal Data for the Public Good: New Opportunities to Enrich Understanding of Individual and Population Health. Calit2, UC Irvine and UC San Diego. Supported by a grant from the Robert Wood Johnson Foundation. Available at http://www.rwjf.org/content/dam/farm/reports/reports/2014/rwjf411080. Accessed 18, 2015.

Hickman, Larry A., and Giuseppe Spadafora. 2009. *John Dewey's Educational Philosophy in International Perspective: A New Democracy for the Twenty-First Century*. Carbondale/Edwardsville: Southern Illinois University Press.

Hood, Leroy, and David Galas. 2003. "The Digital Code of DNA." *Nature* 421 (January 23): 444–448. doi:10.1038/nature01410.

Jackson, Stephen. J., Tarleton Gillespie, and Sandy Payette. 2014. "The Policy Knot: Re-integrating Policy, Practice and Design in CSCW Studies of Social Computing." In *CSCW '14: Proceedings of the 17th ACM conference on Computer Supported Cooperative Work & Social Computing*, 588–602. February 15–19. New York: ACM.

Manovich, Lev. 1998. *Database as a Symbolic Form*. Cambridge, MA: MIT Press.

Manovich, Lev. 2013. "The Algorithms of Our Lives." *The Chronicle of Higher Education*, December 16.

National Commission for the Protection of Human Subjects of Biomedical and Behavioral Research (NCPHS). 1979. "Belmont Report: Ethical Principles and Guidelines for the Protection of Human Subjects of Research." *Federal Register* 44: 23192–23197.

Norberg, P. A., D. R. Horne, and D. A. Horne. 2007. "The Privacy Paradox: Personal Information Disclosure Intentions versus Behaviors." *Journal of Consumer Affairs* 41:100–126. doi:10.1111/j.1745-6606.2006.00070.x.

Quételet, Adolphe. 1869. *Physique Sociale: ou essay sur lé development des facultíes de l'homme*. Brussels: C. Muquardt.

Schüll, Natasha Dow. 2005. "Digital Gambling: The Coincidence of Desire and Design." *Annals of the American Academy of Political and Social Science* 597 (January): 65–81.

Schüll, Natasha Dow. 2012. *Addiction by Design: Machine Gambling in Las Vegas*. Princeton, NJ: Princeton University Press.

Star, Susan Leigh. 1994. "Misplaced Concretism and Concrete Situations: Feminism, Method and Information Technology." Working Paper 11. Gender-Nature-Culture Feminist Research Network: Odense: Odense Universitet, Denmark.

Whitehead, Alfred North. 1925 [1919]. *An Enquiry Concerning the Principles of Natural Knowledge*. 2nd ed. Cambridge, UK and New York: Cambridge University Press.

Whitehead, Alfred North. 1997 [1925]. *Science and the Modern World*. New York: Free Press/Simon & Schuster.

Wild, Christopher. 2005. "Complementing the Genome with an 'Exposome': The Outstanding Challenge of Environmental Exposure Measurement in Molecular Epidemiology." *Cancer Epidemiology, Biomarkers & Prevention: A Publication of the American Association for Cancer Research, Cosponsored by the American Society of Preventive Oncology* 14 (8): 1847–1850.

Wildman, Eugene, and Peter Michelson. 1969 [1967]. *The Chicago Review Anthology of Concretism*. 2nd ed. Chicago: Swallow Press.

# Epilogue

When the research for this book was conceived, only a very small handful of biosensors, in the strict definition, were in use outside of medical settings—ovulation monitors, direct to consumer genomics, and, if you pushed hard enough, as Marc Böhlen did, water-quality sensors. Many researchers instead pursued proxies, like fitness and heart rate monitors, on the theory that they too revealed information about the body and its environment, and could tell us much about the social life of that kind of data. As biosensors become a part of everyday life, they find various preexisting "hooks" to hold onto, often the same hooks that other kinds of sensors also found. Sometimes the hook is legal, such as privacy law that sets the frame for interpreting these new devices in the legal system, while other times it is technical, such as the way sensors are integrated into other hardware and networking systems. The hook can also be within the data themselves, in the ways that designers create or prevent commensurability. When new water-quality biosensors changed the unit of measurement from a spatial one (colony-forming units) to a temporal one (time to detect), the new unit had to be mapped onto the old one in order for the new measurement to be adopted. In still other circumstances, it is ordinary practices like self-tracking that provide the site where biosensors are integrated into everyday life, or rejected.

Biosensors' stories continued to unfold as we wrote this volume, and will continue in the years to come. Although I have suggested that some moments are better than others when trying to steer technology in a different direction, there is no single moment when the technology is finished, once and for all. The volume has refrained from an overall normative prescription for what biosensing should become, but has instead mapped the distinct contours of this emerging, evolving landscape with the goal of enabling readers to intervene where they see fit. In doing so, it has outlined what is destabilizing, and what is being re-entrenched. The ultimate trajectory of these technologies could be yet more biomedicalization, but we have shown that there is ample room to make it otherwise. Making it otherwise could involve building on already viable social dynamics, whether by caring for fellow sufferers, developing new forms of biography and narrative, or turning the clinical gaze inside out. Yet more violations of privacy, and further concentration of control over data might still be in store for us, but this book contains examples of projects that instead create space for more equitable distribution of access and control. It also contains examples of projects that demonstrated, through their actions, care for smaller-scale social relationships, which closes the social distance between the actors such that privacy violations became less of a risk. These projects show that social relations involving biosensors can be done in a respectful way, even in parts of the world where the word "privacy" is not a meaningful concept.

We set out to examine biosensing practices, where sensors reveal something about the body or the environment they are in. It is no small irony, then, that the majority of contributors have found that the boundary between "the body" and "the environment" is being destabilized. Throughout the book this has been a central theme, from the ecological notion of data citizenship, to the recursive notions of self and other, to the ways that "n of 1" can become an "n of a billion 1s." By expanding the range of phenomena that can be electronically sensed and turned into data, biosensors ask people to think twice about the social relations they believe their bodies to be in, and the materials that constitute both those bodies and their ecosystems. It is clear that biosensors do not make anyone's life "simpler," contrary to the claims of product manufacturers. Rather, a biosensor-rich world requires a much more complex notion of where a person's body begins and ends. This destabilization of categories is not unique to the types of biosensing described here, and can be found in other areas of scientific practice. For example, Helmreich's (2008) oceanographers discovered when looking at oceanic microbes that the closer you look, the harder it is to be confident in the categories that distinguish one thing from another. Oceanographers find themselves in an "alien ocean," where it is ever harder to pin down what they thought they were looking for. In a sense, biosensing is a practice where information technology finds alien oceans in the everyday.

Indeed, as we finish our writing, the destabilization of categories is only intensifying. Air quality monitoring and radiation monitoring have become more feasible at both the community and individual level. The environmental justice movement is developing rich datasets, and the substances they measure have everything to do with bodies and health. It is only the conception of the environment as the thing "out there" that prevents air quality data from being linked to personal health data, which supposedly only pertain to "in here." If there is one thing this book demonstrates, it is that data do not just move on their own. The notion of the environment as a kind of externality prevents people from thickening the social, technical, and institutional connections necessary to make data move between those who concern themselves with "health" and those who concern themselves with "the environment." Challenging the notion that body and environment are somehow distinct, as many here have tried to do, would be the first step in making alliances between these two social worlds. It is also only the first step.

Gregory and Bowker use the skin as a way of thinking about the self/environment boundary. Perhaps now that social science has thoroughly denaturalized this boundary, the skin might be worthwhile to contemplate again, as a metaphor for absorption and protection. Both functions matter. Absorption helps us conceive of bodies as part of a wider ecology traceable in data, where barriers are not absolute, and where important connections are to be found. Skin also serves us well as an organ of protection, and this volume has identified many instances where protection is what is needed. At the time of writing, a major fight has broken out over the ownership of data produced by medical implants (noted in chapter 7). People are asking questions about whether the skin is a boundary that *should* trigger some level of dominion over data that is generated underneath the skin. Why, implantees ask, should I not have access to the very data that is produced inside me? Ingestible sensors, which have passed FDA approval, will no doubt raise exactly this question if they are widely adopted. In fact, late night talk show host Stephen Colbert has already satirized the comically tragic prospect of ingestible sensors, which their makers claim will "help patients suffering from diseases of the central nervous system, including schizophrenia ... because nothing is more reassuring to a schizophrenic than a corporation inserting sensors into your body that beam information to all those people watching your every move."[1]

While we can deconstruct notions of self and other all we like, to deny the skin as an important marker of the integrity of the self is downright cruel in this instance. The skin is where implantees draw the boundary between self and nonself, and there is nothing satisfying about yanking the rug out from under them for the sake of theoretical correctness. This raises a question that any serious public discussion of biosensing must address: in what circumstances does it make sense to defend categories like the self as a necessary fiction, and in what circumstances is it better to dispose of them in order to open up a more relational view that allows new categories and communities to flourish, perhaps more equitably than those which came before? Who is best positioned to participate in that flourishing, and who has every incentive to use a newfound relationality to dismiss values that prove inconvenient, or unprofitable? These are questions made possible by social science, but they are not merely intellectual puzzles. They are questions about where care and kindness belong when dealing with unstable categories, and the technologies that destabilize them. Biosensors can be compatible with many different values and beliefs about what makes for human dignity. Some of these values have a more precarious social existence than others, and need more active assertion.

## Note

1. The Colbert Report, "Cheating Death: Sensor Enabled Pills," first aired August 8, 2012, http://thecolbertreport.cc.com/videos/h3tu8s/cheating-death---sensor-enabled-pills---facelift-bungee-cords, accessed July 1, 2015.

## Reference

Helmreich, Stefan. 2008. *Alien Ocean: Anthropological Voyages in Microbial Seas*. Oakland, CA: University of California Press.

# Biographical Sketches

Artist-Engineer **Marc Böhlen** aka RealTechSupport designs speculative machinery that surfaces technical and material challenges, and brings them into real-life existence. His art work has been recognized in awards including the VIDA/ALIFE award (2004) and the VILCEK digital arts award (2013). Böhlen is Professor of Media Study at the University at Buffalo. His work can be found at www.realtechsupport.org.

**Geoffrey C. Bowker** is Professor at the School of Information and Computer Science, University of California at Irvine, where he directs a laboratory for Values in the Design of Information Systems and Technology. Recent positions include Professor of and Senior Scholar in Cyberscholarship at the University of Pittsburgh iSchool and Executive Director, Center for Science, Technology and Society, Santa Clara. Together with Susan Leigh Star Bowker wrote *Sorting Things Out: Classification and Its Consequences*; his most recent book is *Memory Practices in the Sciences*.

**Sophie Day** is Professor of Anthropology at Goldsmiths, London. She is currently working on relations of care in the UK National Health Service as Visiting Professor in the School of Public Health, Imperial College London. Much of her work focuses on health as a lens into "problem spaces," with a particular interest in new methodologies. She has worked in Europe and Ladakh (India) on relations of care, labor, and kinship across the lifecourse.

After six years developing and launching products at Google—from the original Nexus One to the Google Art Project—**Anna de Paula Hanika** returned to her passion for innovating in health at Open mHealth, leading product strategy and marketing. She studied neurophysiology and experimental psychology at Oxford University, UK.

**Deborah Estrin** is a Professor of Computer Science at Cornell Tech in New York City and a Professor of Public Health at Weill Cornell Medical College. She is founder of the Healthier Life Hub and directs the Small Data Lab at Cornell Tech, which develops new personal data APIs and applications for individuals to harvest the small data traces they generate daily. Estrin is also cofounder of the nonprofit startup, Open mHealth.

**Brittany Fiore-Gartland** is a postdoctoral fellow in the eScience Institute and the Department of Human-Centered Design and Engineering at the University of Washington working as a data science ethnographer. Her research focuses on the social and organizational dimensions of data-intensive transformations in arenas such as scientific research, health care, global development, and design and construction. Using an ethnographic approach, she explores the challenges and opportunities for communication and collaboration during moments of technological change.

**Dana Greenfield**, PhD, is a medical student in the MD/PhD program at UC San Francisco, where she also earned her doctorate from the Joint Program in Medical Anthropology (UCSF/UC Berkeley) in 2015. She received her BA from Barnard College, Columbia University, in Anthropology and Biology. Her work takes an ethnographic approach to understanding the socio-cultural implications of digital health technologies and personal health data.

**Judith Gregory** is a Co-Director of the EVOKE & Values in Design of Information Systems and Technology Laboratory, Informatics, University of California at Irvine. She has long been concerned with personal genomics and more recently with Quantified Self technologies related to themes of "Living Algorithmically" and "Privacy and Trust."

**Mette Kragh-Furbo** is a PhD candidate in the Department of Sociology at Lancaster University, UK. Her work focuses on personal genomics as practice and its entanglements with digital culture and experimentation. She is interested in socio-cultural issues of biomedicine and the social life of health data. She works at the intersections of science and technology studies, sociology of health and illness, and digital culture.

**Celia Lury** is Director of the Centre for Interdisciplinary Methodologies, University of Warwick. Her recent research is concerned with the ways in which "live" methods enact social worlds. Current investigations involve looking the role of methods: in brand valuation, ranking influence in social media, tracking and surveillance, and personalization. Recent publications include *Inventive Methods* (coedited with Nina Wakeford, Routledge, 2012), *Measure and Value* (coedited with Lisa Adkins, Blackwell, 2012), and a Special Issue of *Theory, Culture and Society* on "Topologies of Culture" (coedited with Luciana Parisi and Tatiana Trinova).

**Adrian Mackenzie** (Professor in Technological Cultures, Department of Sociology, Lancaster University) has published work on technology: *Transductions: Bodies and Machines at Speed* (2006 [2002]), *Cutting Code: Software and Sociality* (2006), and *Wirelessness: Radical Empiricism in Network Cultures* (2010). He is currently working on an archeology of machine learning and its associated transformations. He codirects the Centre for Science Studies, Lancaster University, UK.

**Rajiv Mehta** leads strategy and design consultancy Bhageera Inc, and is an expert in family caregiving, consumer health, and emerging health technologies. He has led pioneering research on family caregiving, and the development of innovative consumer technologies. Earlier, he modeled atmospheric turbulence at NASA, sparked the digital camera revolution at Apple, and led innovation for Adobe, Symbol, and numerous startups. Mehta is a board member, Family Caregiver Alliance, and co-organizer, Quantified Self. He holds degrees from Columbia (MBA), Stanford (MS), and Princeton (BSE).

**Maggie Mort** is Professor in the Sociology of Science, Technology, and Medicine, Lancaster University, UK. She coordinated the EC FP7 Science in Society project, Ethical Frameworks for Telecare Technologies for older people at home (EFORTT). She teaches and supervises in disaster studies, health policy and practice, patient safety, and medical uncertainty. She has published widely on technological change, most recently in health care, and on technological legitimations of public policy in defense, medicine, social care, and emergency planning.

**Dawn Nafus** is a Senior Research Scientist at Intel Labs, where she conducts anthropological research to inspire new products and services. She has published widely on experiences of time, gender and technology, ethnography in industry, and most recently, quantification. With Lama Nachman, she also co-led the Data Sense project, which created data processing and visualization tools for nonexpert use (www.makesenseofdata.com). She is the co-author of *Self-Tracking* (MIT Press 2016) with Gina Neff. She holds a PhD from the University of Cambridge.

**Gina Neff** is associate professor of communication at the University of Washington. She is author of *Venture Labor* (MIT Press 2012) and with Dawn Nafus *Self-Tracking* (MIT Press 2016). With Carrie Sturts Dossick she codirects the Collaboration, Technology and Organizational Practices research group that studies how construction teams work together with data for better buildings. Her research has been funded by the National Science Foundation, Intel, and Microsoft Research.

**Helen Nissenbaum,** Professor of Media, Culture, and Communication and Director of the Information Law Institute at New York University, is author and editor of seven books, including *Obfuscation: A User's Guide for Privacy and Protest*, with Finn Brunton (MIT Press 2015). Privacy has been a central focus of her research, alongside big data, bias in computer systems, politics of search engines, accountability, values in design, and other issues in the societal dimensions of information technologies.

**Heather Patterson** is a cognitive scientist and legal scholar who investigates how people conceptualize and manage privacy and information flows when navigating emerging socio-technological systems. She is a Senior Research Scientist at Intel Labs and an Affiliate Scholar at New York University's Information Law Institute.

**Celia Roberts** is the Co-Director of the Centre for Gender and Women's Studies and Senior Lecturer in Sociology at Lancaster University. She works on sex and sexuality, health technologies, and aging and feminist theory, and is the author of *Puberty in Crisis: The Sociology of Sexual Development* (Cambridge University Press 2015).

**Jamie Sherman** is a cultural anthropologist (PhD Princeton) and research scientist at Intel Corporation. Her research background is in techniques and technologies of self-transformation, inequality, and the body. Since joining Intel in 2012, her work has focused on emerging technology objects and practices including wearable technologies, personal data tracking, and relational computing.

**Alex Taylor** is a sociologist working at Microsoft Research Cambridge. He has undertaken investigations into a range of routine and often mundane aspects of everyday life. For instance, he's developed what some might see as an unhealthy preoccupation with hoarding, dirt, clutter, and similar seemingly banal subject matter. Most recently, he's begun obsessing over computation and wondering what the compulsion for seeing-data-everywhere might mean for the future of humans and machines. His work can be found at http://ast.io and the twitter handle @alx_tylr.

**Gary Wolf** is the cofounder of the Quantified Self, a global collaboration among users and makers of self-tracking tools exploring "self-knowledge through numbers." Wolf is also a contributing editor at *Wired* magazine. His work has appeared in *The Best American Science Writing* (2009) and in *The Best American Science and Nature Writing* (2009). In 2010, he was awarded the AAAS Kavli Science Journalism prize. In 2005–2006 he was a John S. Knight Fellow at Stanford University.

# Index

Note: italicized page numbers denote figures.

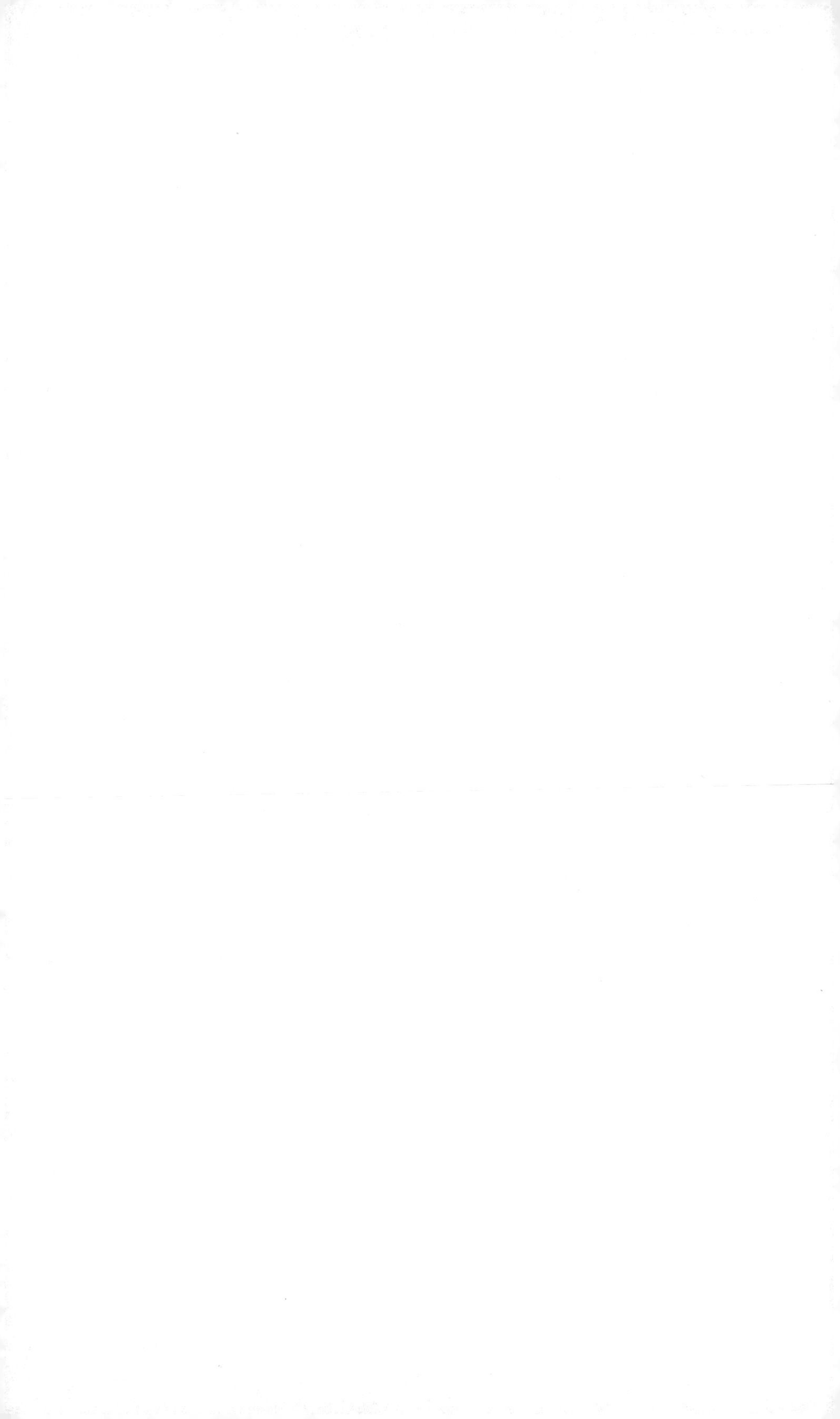